PELICAN BOOKS

A 456

EPIDEMIC DISEASES

A. H. GALE

EPIDEMIC DISEASES

A. H. GALE

PENGUIN BOOKS

Penguin Books Ltd, Harmondsworth, Middlesex
U.S.A.: Penguin Books Inc., 3300 Clipper Mill Road, Baltimore 11, Md
AUSTRALIA: Penguin Books Pty Ltd, 762 Whitehorse Road,
Mitcham, Victoria

—

First published 1959

—

Made and printed in Great Britain
by Spottiswoode, Ballantyne & Co. Ltd
London and Colchester

CONTENTS

LIST OF FIGURES

FOREWORD

THIS book on pestilence through the ages was almost completed when Arthur Gale died so prematurely in 1956. I was asked by Mrs Gale to edit the volume, a task which I gladly accepted and which has given me great personal pleasure.

The work has not proved easy as, although conversant with much of the book since its conception, I had little knowledge of the sources to which Arthur Gale had turned to compile this fund of knowledge.

I should like to express my thanks to Professor Bruce Perry for much helpful advice, and for writing the preface to this work. Also to John Lane, The Bodley Head Ltd, for permission to include certain plates and diagrams contained in a book by Walter G. Bell, F.S.A., F.R.A.S., entitled *The Great Plague of London in 1665* and published by The Bodley Head.

E. R. HARGREAVES

PREFACE

When Dr Arthur Gale died in October 1956 he left the nearly completed manuscript of this book which represents an expression of the main guiding interest of his professional life. The changes in the epidemiology of the common infectious diseases had interested him for many years. Always keenly interested in the welfare of children, he was, from 1933 to 1947, one of the medical officers to the Board of Education. Some of his researches during this time formed the basis of his Milroy Lectures to the Royal College of Physicians in 1944 on 'A Century of Changes in the Mortality and Incidence of the Principal Infections of Childhood'. His increasing interest in epidemiology lead in 1947 to his transfer to the Ministry of Health. There he became a member of the epidemiological team and was thus enabled to continue his studies on the epidemiological features of acute anterior poliomyelitis. In 1950 he was invited by the University of Bristol to accept the combined posts of Director of Medical Post-Graduate Studies and Lecturer in Epidemiology. The former post brought him into contact with consultants and practitioners throughout the West Country, and this enabled him, with their help, to continue his researches. He was particularly intrigued by the way in which epidemics of anterior poliomyelitis widely separated in time struck the same villages in the south-west, and he spent much time and thought in attempting to solve this problem. This book, written in simple and non-technical terms, introduces to the layman the fascinating history of the common infectious diseases in this country. After Dr Gale's death the manuscript has been completed and in a few places brought up to date by one of his great friends, Dr E. R. Hargreaves, Deputy Medical Officer for the County of Cornwall. It is largely due to Dr Hargreaves's enthusiasm and devoted care in preparing the manuscript that the book is now published. It forms a most fitting memorial to Dr Gale's life-work.

C. Bruce Perry, M.D., F.R.C.P.

INTRODUCTION

THERE are many books on the history of medicine and several on the history of public health, but the only book which deals systematically with the history of epidemic diseases in this country is Creighton's great work of scholarship, *The History of Epidemics in Britain*, published in two volumes in 1894. Creighton's book is an inexhaustible store of information, but it is not the kind of book which anyone would read unless he had a special interest in the subject. Greenwood's *Epidemics and Crowd Diseases* is the nearest approach to a history for the general reader, but the first part of it is concerned with the development of epidemiological theory from the time of Hippocrates, and the second treats of individual diseases as examples to illustrate epidemiological principles. Thus Greenwood's book is in some ways more comprehensive than this one and in others less. He ranges the world for his examples, but he does not include all the epidemic diseases which have at some time been important in Britain.

In an address to the National Book League, Trevelyan once said: 'Besides the contemplation and study of the past for its own sake, there remains the second great value of history, namely, the light it throws on the present.' There can be little doubt about the intrinsic interest of the history of epidemic diseases, but there may be some about the value of this study for the light it throws upon the present because many of the diseases to be discussed have vanished from the English scene or have become trivial. However, infantile paralysis is still with us; we can never be quite sure what influenza may do, and several of the other diseases cause a great deal of sickness even if they no longer kill as they used to do.

The chief criterion for the inclusion of a disease has been that it has at some time been epidemic in the dictionary sense of being prevalent at one time and not at another. Some diseases which are certainly epidemic, for example

13

chicken-pox and mumps, have perforce been omitted because they have led such blameless lives from the point of view of causing serious damage that they have little recorded history.

All the diseases to be discussed are believed to be due to micro-organisms, and, although my aim has been to write a book which shall be intelligible to the general reader, it is hardly possible to avoid the use of some technical terms in writing about them.

Each chapter begins with a short summary of modern knowledge about the disease or diseases to be discussed, but the following general remarks may help the non-technical reader to understand these summaries. Most of the micro-organisms which cause important epidemic diseases in human beings in Britain belong to two main classes: (1) the bacteria, or (2) the viruses. The bacteria belong to a world in which the unit of measurement is the micron, i.e. one thousandth of a millimetre – written 1μ. They are visible directly under the highest power of an ordinary microscope. The viruses belong to a world in which the unit of measurement is only one thousandth of 1μ – written $1 m\mu$ – but they vary in size more than the bacteria, the largest of them being about $300 m\mu$ in length or diameter, whereas the smallest are about $10–20 m\mu$. The largest viruses may be just visible under the highest power of an ordinary microscope, but most of them can be made visible only in photographs taken with an electron microscope. Bacteria can multiply outside the body and are habitually grown in enormous numbers in or on various substances in thousands of bacteriological laboratories throughout the world. Viruses, though they can survive outside the animal body, cannot multiply except within living cells, and so, in laboratories, they have to be grown either in fertile living eggs or in a living culture of animal tissue. This is obviously a more difficult and limiting technique than that of the culture of bacteria in a culture medium composed of broth or agar or some similar substance. All animal diseases due to micro-organisms may be regarded as the reaction of a host to a parasite, the animal being the host and the micro-organism the parasite. The epidemic process is fundamentally the same as that which the gardener sees when his strawberry plants or his raspberry canes proceed to die off from a virus infection.

Animals, including man, have a highly complex mechanism for protecting themselves against attack by micro-organisms and producing immunity, and the following scheme gives some idea of how this works:

$$\text{Immunity} \begin{cases} \text{Innate} \\ \text{Acquired} \begin{cases} \text{Passive} \\ \text{Active} \end{cases} \end{cases}$$

Not very much is known about innate immunity, but it obviously exists, because some micro-organisms have power to produce disease in many different kinds of animals whereas others affect only one kind. It seems possible that there may be genetic differences between individual human beings which determine, to some extent, their susceptibility to different diseases, but we have little exact knowledge about this.

Acquired immunity is dependent on the fact that the introduction of the parasite into the host results in the production of protective substances. The substances in the parasite which provoke this response are known as antigens, and the substances produced by the host are called antibodies. The details of antigen–antibody reactions in special cases are extremely complicated, and a large proportion of the time of bacteriologists is spent in working out such details, but for our purpose it is sufficient to know that antigen provokes the production of antibody, that a single micro-organism may incorporate a number of different antigens, and that variations in the antigenic structure of some micro-organisms frequently occur both under natural conditions and in the laboratory.

We speak of immunity as being active when the host has itself manufactured antibodies as a result of invasion by a parasite, and we speak of it as passive when some other host has done the manufacturing and the ready-made antibodies are transferred from this host to the one we wish to protect. Active immunity may occur naturally as a result of infection or be produced artificially by the administration of some form of protective vaccine, a vaccine being a suspension of complete or part micro-organisms, alive or dead, the suspension thus containing antigens which, when inoculated, will stimulate the production of antibodies in the susceptible person. Passive immunity may occur naturally, when antibodies pass from the mother to her unborn child, or it may be produced artificially by the administration of blood serum to an animal which has no antibody from one which has. Passive immunity tends to be a temporary affair, and in this book the words immunization and immunity may be taken to imply the active process unless the passive one is specifically mentioned.

In practice there are great differences between the efficacy of different vaccines. Bacteriologists are always striving to find antigens which are harmless in themselves but will produce a large amount of antibody against the particular micro-organism concerned, and they have had to use many different methods to protect against different diseases. Sometimes the antigen is a harmless (or almost harmless) strain of living virus, for example the vaccine used to protect against smallpox; sometimes it is an extract made from virulent bacteria made harmless by the addition of a chemical, for example diphtheria prophylactic; sometimes it is a suspension of killed bacteria, for example whooping-cough vaccine. In the study of individual diseases we shall find one, diphtheria, whose history seems to have been affected profoundly by artificial immunization; one, smallpox, in which the part played by immunization is difficult to assess; and many whose history has so far been unaffected. We have to remember that the process of natural immunization goes on all the time. Sometimes it is obvious, as in a community of young children which suffers an epidemic of measles and then remains free from the disease until there are enough unimmunized recruits to provide fuel for another epidemic. Sometimes it is less obvious because the presence of some micro-organisms in a community may produce a great deal of immunity without producing much overt disease. In this respect the history of the disease is an imperfect reflection of the reaction between the community and its parasites.

Another factor which has profoundly affected the history of these epidemic diseases is that of the mechanism of their transmission from one host to another. The mechanism of infection is sometimes a complicated one, involving animal and insect intermediaries as vectors. Thus the incidence of disease in man may be determined not only by the prevalence of the parasite and man's susceptibility to it, but also by the ecology of the intermediate host or hosts. On this line of thought there is a theory that the disappearance of plague from Europe towards the end of the seventeenth century was largely due to the replacement of the black rat by the brown, and this explanation is often quoted in history books. There is, however, one great difficulty in accepting the theory, and this will be discussed later.

Finally, we have to consider changes in the parasite. There are numerous examples of diseases which have undoubtedly changed their behaviour in a way which suggests that the causal organism has changed. Sometimes the change has been a sudden one, for example, when influenza caused such devastation in 1918–19 or when mild smallpox first appeared, and sometimes there has been a gradual change, as exemplified by the history of scarlet fever. We know little about these changes in nature, but we know that in the laboratory bacteria and viruses may change their virulence considerably. Generally speaking, if a bacterial culture is kept going in a laboratory for some time the organism tends to lose virulence, whereas if it is passed through a series of animals the bacteria tend to gain virulence. Some of the recent work of Burnet* on the changes in influenza virus when grown in the laboratory in fertile hen's eggs is most intriguing from the epidemiological point of view.

We must remember that all bacteriological knowledge is historically new. Before about 1880 the only way of classifying diseases was by their signs and symptoms, and classification founded on the identification of the micro-organism came late and did not always coincide with the older classification. For this reason many chapters begin with a description of the history of some rather vague groups of diseases,

* F. M. Burnet, 1944.

for example the 'continued fevers', and then branch out into a description of the diseases which probably made up that group. The modern classification did not always have to wait for the discovery of the causal organism, because clinical differentiation was proceeding apace before the discovery of bacteria, but bacteriology has, nevertheless, produced a revolution in modes of thought about communicable diseases.

It is much easier to write the history of a disease which has characteristic signs and symptoms, such as plague, than of one which has indefinite signs and symptoms, such as influenza. But many diseases can be identified in the ancient records from the combined study of their clinical and epidemiological characteristics.

I

AN EXAMINATION OF SOURCES

It is necessary to begin with a rather protracted examination of sources, because in medicine, perhaps more than in any other subject, ideas and nomenclature have changed enormously even in the last seventy years and almost out of recognition between 1348 and 1950.

For the earliest period, from 1348 to the reign of Henry VIII (1509–47), we depend for information chiefly on monastic histories, state documents, and, for the Black Death, on the rolls of manor courts. There are also many fragmentary references to epidemics in letters of the time. Medical books begin to be useful in the Tudor Period and become continuously more so from the time of the great physicians of the Commonwealth and Restoration – Sydenham, Willis, and Morton.

In the Tudor Period also there were the beginnings of statistical records in the London Bills of Mortality (see Appendix, p. 149) and the parish registers. As these will be mentioned frequently when the history of individual diseases is discussed, a little more may be said about them.

The London Bills of Mortality began, probably, in 1532, and the first of them which is extant tells 'how many syns the 17th day of November until the 23rd day of the same month is dead within the city and freedom young and old these many following of the plague and other diseases'. This Bill accounts for only sixty-six deaths and is almost certainly incomplete. In the next thirty years the Bills were issued irregularly, probably only when plague was epidemic, but between 1563 and 1592 the regular series began. It is not clear how the first Bills were compiled, but early in their history they became the responsibility of the Company of Parish Clerks. This Company was granted a royal charter in the thirteenth century and its function was connected with church music. When a rich citizen died, the whole company might be engaged to sing at his funeral, and thus it acquired the apparently incongruous function of registering births and deaths. By 1581 the procedure had become formal. In every parish two 'discrete' matrons were selected to be searchers. They were sworn before the Dean of Arches at the Church of St Mary le Bow to 'search the body of every such person as shall happen to die in the same parish and to report weekly to the parish clerk'. The parish clerk had to make a weekly report to the warden of the parish clerks, who sent it to the mayor, who sent it to the minister of state. The purpose of the Bills was to warn the great ones of the court and of the city when plague was about so that they might depart in good time for the purer air of the countryside.

In 1625 the Company obtained a decree of Star Chamber permitting them to set up a special printing press for the issue of weekly and annual Bills. At first, numbers of burials from plague and from all other causes, and numbers of christenings were returned. In 1629 causes of death other than plague were distinguished, and the totals of deaths from all causes were separated by sex. In 1727 the ages of those dying were given, and in this form the Bills continued until 1849, eleven years after the establishment of the General Register Office had made them obsolete. In 1955 the weekly return of the Registrar-General still includes a memento of the Bills, for Table III of the report is a return of the deaths, by age, sex, and cause, registered in London during the week.

For places outside London, the sources of information about births, deaths, and sometimes causes of death are the parish registers. These were kept with different degrees of care in different places from the reign of Elizabeth. One of the inaccuracies of the Bills of Mortality and of the parish registers is that they did not include the deaths of Dissenters.

There are then two main streams of information about the incidence and mortality of disease from the middle of the seventeenth century. One is medical literature, which was contributed largely by the fashionable physicians in London and makes little use of figures, and the other is the incomplete information in the Bills and parish registers. At first the physicians made no use of the Bills, and indeed they probably held them in contempt because they were based on the diagnoses of ignorant women. It was left to a business-man called John Graunt* (1620–74) to make the first serious study of the despised Bills. His *Observations on the Bills of Mortality* are generally regarded as the first important con-tribution to the study of vital statistics ever made, and his handling of the extremely inadequate material at his disposal was masterly. He knew that he was on much safer ground in making deductions from total numbers of deaths than in using information about deaths from individual causes, and some of the principles he adopted in analysing the Bills are still of first-rate importance to anyone who tries to draw con-clusions from figures of deaths by cause. These principles seem simple, but it is surprising how often they have been and still are forgotten. When Graunt found that deaths from a certain cause seemed to be increasing in the Bills over a period of years he was always careful to scrutinize the figures of deaths from nearly related causes to make sure that deaths from the cause he was examining really had increased, and that the increase was not an artefact due to a change in classification or nomenclature. In plague years he found that it was not only deaths from plague which increased, but also those from many other causes, and he suspected that deaths from plague were being concealed because of the inconveni-ence which a death from plague in a house might cause to the other inmates. Perhaps some of the discrepancies were due not to deliberate concealment but to genuine mistakes, for a similar phenomenon is seen today in years of epidemic influenza.

This seems very simple and obvious, but two examples may be given to show that the importance of scrutinizing sources was and is sometimes overlooked. When examining the Bills of a later period, William Heberden the younger† concluded that deaths from dysentery had declined marked-ly. He assumed that 'griping of the guts' in the Bills was synonymous with dysentery. In fact it was what we call 'infantile diarrhoea' and the deaths from it had merely to

* John Graunt, 1662.　　　　　† William Heberden, 1813.

be transferred to the heading 'convulsions'. The second example is rather different, but also illustrates the importance of knowing one's sources. It is taken from an article by Bradford Hill*:

In the course of a single committee meeting I have heard a distinguished surgeon reject as quite valueless the death certificates obtained in a follow-up of patients with cancer and yet express the greatest interest in the cancer mortality data by site of growth published by the Registrar-General. He apparently saw no inconsistency in this attitude towards material obtained from precisely the same sources, and such an attitude is by no means rare.

Up to 1839 the Bills of parish registers were the only continuous records of births and deaths, but in certain places quite good records were kept for restricted periods. For Carlisle, for example, there are records of deaths by age and cause for the years 1779–87 (omitting the year 1780). In 1750 Dr Thomas Short published his *New observations, Natural, Moral, Civil, Political, and Medical, on City, Town, and Country Bills of Mortality*. As the title suggests, this is a discursive book but it does contain many abstracts of the registers of parishes for a long period of years.

In 1801 the first decennial census was taken, so that for the first time reasonably accurate and comprehensive figures of population became available. In July 1837 national registration of births and deaths began, and in 1839 Samuel Farr was appointed to be compiler of abstracts at the new General Register Office. For the first time comprehensive, though at first incomplete, information about fatal diseases became available for the country as a whole. In his nomenclature of fatal diseases for statistical purposes, Farr divided them into two main groups: (1) Epidemic, endemic, and contagious diseases; (2) Sporadic diseases. We are concerned with those diseases in group 1, and Farr's list is much more intelligible to the modern reader than are the names used in the Bills. The changes in nomenclature since Farr's time have been evolutionary rather than revolutionary. There are two important omissions from Farr's list: diphtheria and

* A. Bradford Hill, 1947.

typhoid fever. Deaths from diphtheria were included under scarlatina or possibly under one of the other headings for diseases of the throat until 1885, and typhoid was included with typhus until 1869. Statistics of the incidence of diseases came much later than those of deaths. For some large cities the number of notifications of certain infectious diseases has been collected since 1898, but for the whole country the series began in 1911 and from time to time new diseases were added. For example, poliomyelitis was added in 1912, encephalitis lethargica in 1918, measles and whooping-cough in 1940.

The great physicians of the Commonwealth and Restoration, of whom Sydenham is the outstanding example, made important contributions to the clinical differentiation of diseases, and so some contribution to the study of their prevalence and fatality at different times. It must be remembered, however, that for the most part they practised in London and among the well-to-do classes, so that they probably knew little about the diseases of the poor, which bulked so large in the Bills, and even less about the diseases of the countryside. In the eighteenth century the founding of voluntary hospitals and of public dispensaries brought medical men of distinction into much closer contact with the poor of the cities, and some of their writings are valuable to the student of the history of diseases. Towards the end of the eighteenth century fever hospitals began to be established, and their records are a useful supplement to the statistics which the office of the Registrar-General began to collect in 1837. One of the results of the sanitary reforms of the period 1848–60 was the establishment of local and central departments of health. The first medical officer of the central department was Sir John Simon,* who early set about the task of collecting and analysing information about the incidence and fatality of epidemic diseases in different parts of the country. An early example of the sort of inquiry he promoted was that of Dr E.H. Greenhow† into deaths by cause in different districts of England and Wales. From 1858

* Sir John Simon, 1856.
† E. H. Greenhow.

to 1872 Simon was medical officer to the Privy Council, and during that period he promoted inquiries into the prevalence and distribution of epidemic diseases, which have served as models for the many official reports since written. His reports and those of his successors are necessarily the chief source from which the history of diseases in the last hundred years has been written.

2

PLAGUE

PLAGUE is due to a bacillus (*Pasteurella pestis*) which can cause disease in man and in many animals, among which rodents and particularly rats are the most important. The commonest form of the human disease is bubonic plague, which begins as an epizootic or glandular infection among rats and reaches man through the bites of rat-fleas which have deserted their normal host after its death. Occasionally plague occurs in man as a deadly form of pneumonia, and this form can spread directly from man to man through the air.

There have been three pandemics of plague in the last 1,500 years. The first was that which came with the corn ships from Egypt and Byzantium in the reign of Justinian in 542–3, the second was the Black Death which reached England in 1348, and the third began in 1894. We do not know whether the Justinian plague reached England, as the chronicles of the time are not sufficiently precise to make identification of pestilences possible. The Black Death is singled out by Trevelyan* as the unique disaster of English social history, and after it plague persisted in England for three hundred years. The latest pandemic affected England not at all in a dramatic sense, but certain events probably associated with it are of great interest to the epidemiologist.

The Black Death has been taken as the starting point of this book because it is one of the outstanding events of world history and because it is the first epidemic, in Britain, of a disease which we can identify with certainty.

Nothing is known for certain of the remote place of origin of the Black Death, but it seems fairly well established that the immediate source of infection for Europe was the Crimea.

* G. M. Trevelyan, 1942.

The eyewitnesses' account given by de Mussis and summarized by Creighton* is a convincing one.

The substance of this story is that the Italian merchants who were then settled in considerable numbers at the various termini or entrepôts of the overland trade from China and Central Asia by the more northern route, were harassed by the Tartar hordes; that they had stood a siege in Tana, on the Don, but had been driven out of it, and had sought refuge for themselves and their merchandise within the walls of Caffa, a small fortified post on the Crimean Straits (of Kertch), built by Genoese not long before; that Caffa was besieged in due course by the Tartar barbarians; that the investment lasted nearly three years; that the merchants and others crowded into the narrow space within the walls were put to great straits and could hardly breathe, being only partially relieved by the arrival of a ship with supplies; that the plague broke out among the besieging Tartar host and daily destroyed thousands; that the Tartars threw the pestilent dead bodies inside the walls by their engines of siege, so that the infection took hold of those within the fort; that the Tartars dispersed in panic and spread the infection all over the shores of the Euxine, Caspian, and Levant; that such of the Italian traders as were able, de Mussis himself with them, escaped from Caffa in a ship; and that the infection appeared in Genoa in its most deadly form a day or two after the arrival of the ship, although none of those on board were suffering from the plague.

Plague probably arrived in England at Weymouth (then Melcombe) at the beginning of August 1348. It is said to have spread rapidly through Dorset, Devon, and Somerset, and to have reached Bristol sometime in August. From Bristol it came to Gloucester, from Gloucester to Oxford, and from Oxford to London, which it reached by 1 November. The Eastern Counties and the north, which suffered very severely, were attacked rather later – probably in the spring and summer of 1349. By the winter of 1349 the Black Death was over, but epidemic plague was established in England and was destined to recur in many lesser but still great epidemics until its final disappearance in 1665-6.

It is, of course, impossible to arrive at any exact figure of the total mortality from the Black Death, but by piecing together scraps of information from all kinds of sources histor-

* C. Creighton, 1894.

ians have concluded that probably a quarter and possibly one-third of the inhabitants of England died of plague in the years 1348-9. Some idea of the prevailing sense of desolation and despair is contained in the following quotation from the chronicle of an Irish friar (quoted by Creighton*):

And I, Friar John Clyn of the Order of Friars Minor, and of the convent of Kilkenny, wrote in this book those notable things which happened in my time, which I saw with my eyes, or which I learned from persons worthy of credit. And lest things worthy of remembrance should perish with time, and fall away from the memory of those who are to come after us, I, seeing these many evils, and the whole world lying, as it were, in the wicked one, among the dead waiting for death till it came – as I have truly heard and examined, so have I reduced these things to writing; and lest the writing should perish with the writer, and the work fail together with the workman, I leave parchment for continuing the work, if haply any man survive and any of the race of Adam escape this pestilence and continue the work which I have commenced.

Most of the contemporary monastic chronicles are, however, interrupted in 1348-9, and if there is an entry under the year 1349, it consists merely of the words '*magna mortalitas*'. One can only imagine that one chronicler was prevented by death from continuing his task and another could find no words to describe so terrible a calamity.

The characteristic which distinguished the Black Death from later outbreaks of plague was more its universal distribution than its high mortality in individual places. It caused devastation in remote places and in the towns, whereas early in its subsequent history plague became a disease particularly of the towns and of the poorer inhabitants of them. London was much larger than any other town, probably having a population of about forty thousand, compared with the six or seven thousand of Bristol or Norwich. Much of our information about plague after the Black Death is contained in state documents concerning the movements of the court, letters of ambassadors, and the like. For these reasons London occupies a prominent place in the history of outbreaks after the Black Death. The identification of these outbreaks is

* C. Creighton, 1894.

not always easy, because the word *pestis* was sometimes used in a generic sense and was not confined to bubonic plague.

After the Black Death there were probably four or five considerable outbreaks of plague before the end of the fourteenth century. They occurred in 1361, 1368–9, 1375, and 1390–1. There is also some record of a severe epidemic in 1381–2 which may or may not have been plague. In the fifteenth century the first great outburst was in 1406–7, and there were major epidemics in London in 1464, 1479, and 1500. Between these major outbreaks, however, there are many records of lesser ones which were sufficiently important to justify the prorogation of Parliament (for example in 1433 and 1437).

The story of plague in the sixteenth century is very like that in the fifteenth. Except for a period of quiescence in the reigns of Edward VI (1547–53) and Mary (1553–8) the disease was nearly always present in London and there were great outbursts in 1500, 1513, 1563, 1569, and 1593.

The first extant Bill of Mortality is assigned with probability to the year 1532, and from 1563 one can begin to construct a continuous if incomplete picture of the annual mortalities from the disease in London. Figure 2 shows the number of deaths from plague in the London Bills from 1563 to 1666. In spite of their defects, the Bills give some idea of the relative importance of plague to Londoners. In the four non-plague years 1597–1600 the Bills showed an average of about 4,250 burials and 4,500 baptisms each year, in other words an excess of births over deaths of 1,000 for the four years. In 1603 plague was credited with 33,347 deaths in London (other years over 10,000). When these figures are considered in relation to one another it is easy to see why those of our ancestors who were in a position to do so moved hastily to the country when plague was about. In this period also there are many accounts of plague in the provinces associated particularly with the movements of armies in the Civil War. An example is the outbreak in Bristol in 1645 at the time of the siege of Prince Rupert's army by that of Fairfax. It is said that there were 3,000 deaths in the city.

The great plague of 1665 is, thanks to Defoe* and Pepys†, almost as well known an event in English history as the Black Death. It is difficult to compare its mortality with that of previous outbreaks because we do not know for certain the number of deaths or the population. Creighton‡, however, gives the following table of comparison between the mortalities from plague in London (including the liberties and out-parishes) in 1603, 1625, and 1665:

Year	Estimated population	Total number of deaths	Number of deaths from plague	Largest number of deaths in a week	Worst week
1603	250,000	42,940	33,347	3,385	25 Aug.–1 Sept.
1625	320,000	63,001	41,313	5,205	11 Aug.–18 Aug.
1665	460,000	97,306	68,596	8,297	12 Sept.–19 Sept.

In the County of London today, with a population of nearly 3½ million, the usual number of deaths in a week in winter is round about 1,000.

Although Defoe was only about six years old in 1665, and we do not know whether he was in London, he used the best contemporary authorities in compiling his *Journal of the Plague Year*. He wrote it in 1722 when plague had acquired a particular 'news' value because of the epidemic in Marseille and Provence which was the last great outbreak in western Europe. Pepys makes frequent references to plague, some of which are worth quoting because they show how the calamity affected a distinguished civil servant.

June 7th, 1665. This day much against my will, I did in Drury Lane see two or three houses marked with a red cross on the doors, and 'Lord have mercy on us' writ there; which was a sad sight to me, being the first of the kind that, to my remembrance, I ever saw. It put me into an ill conception of myself and to my smell, so that I was forced to buy some roll-tobacco to smell and to chaw which took away the apprehension.

June 29th. Up and by water to White Hall, where the court full of waggons and people ready to go out of town.

* D. Defoe, 1722. † S. Pepys, 1825.
‡ C. Creighton, 1894.

July 10th. An unpleasing thing to be at Court, everybody being fearful one of another.

August 30th. Met with Hadley, our clerke for, says he, there died 9 this week, tho' I have returned but 6 which is a very ill practice and makes me think it is so in other places; and therefore the plague much greater than people take it to be.

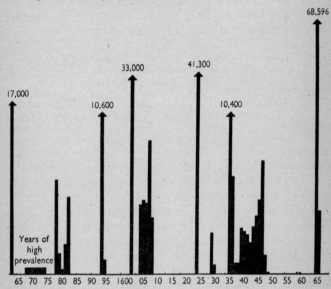

1. *Annual deaths from plague recorded in the London Bills of Mortality between 1563 and 1666*

The last extract is an interesting commentary on the changes in the structure of society since Pepys's time. It is difficult to imagine a casual conversation in Whitehall today between the registrar for the City of Westminster and the permanent secretary of the Admiralty in the course of which the registrar mentioned to the permanent secretary that he had just falsified his weekly return to the Registrar-General!

Although statistical information about the plague of 1665 is admittedly inaccurate, it does enable us to form a reasonably clear picture of the main facts about its incidence and spread. Figures 1–5 illustrate the main facts. Figure 2 shows

the deaths returned in the weekly Bills from January 1665
to March 1666. Both the total number of deaths and the
number of deaths from plague are shown and it is obvious
that whereas at the beginning of the year some five hundred
deaths were returned every week, at the height of the epidemic in August and September over 8,000 a week were
returned for all causes and about 7,000 from plague. It appears therefore that there may have been some 500 more
deaths from plague in a week than were shown in the returns.
The quotation from Pepys's diary supports this view.

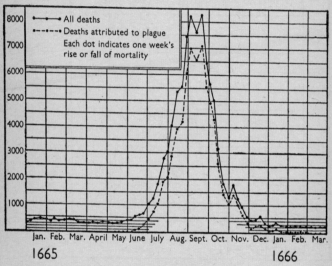

2. *Deaths from plague and other causes returned in the Bills of Mortality for 1665–6*

Figure 3 shows how the plague spread from west to east.
The position of the parishes (St Giles, Cripplegate, and Stepney) is indicated in Figure 4, which also shows how the City
itself escaped relatively lightly when compared with the
Liberties and Out-parishes. At this time the City was still
the home of the prosperous merchants, and the poor lived
for the most part in the maze of alleys and courts outside
the walls. The standard of housing was worse here than in
the City itself. The highest mortality of all was in the populous

suburbs of Cripplegate, Whitechapel, Stepney, St Martin-in-the-Fields, St Giles-in-the-Fields, Southwark, and West-minster. Further references will be made to this point when the possible effects of the Great Fire of 1666 are considered.

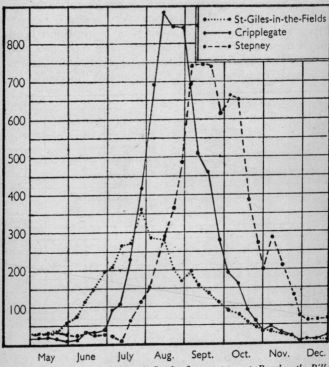

3. *Chart showing trend of plague in London from west to east. Based on the Bills of Mortality for 1665*

On the whole the plague of 1665–6 affected London far more than the provinces, but certain provincial towns had severe outbreaks, notably Yarmouth (November 1664), the eastern counties generally (in 1665–6), and many coast towns in Kent, particularly naval stations (in 1666). There was plague also at Derby and in Derbyshire, and the story of the outbreak at the little isolated village of Eyam in the Peak

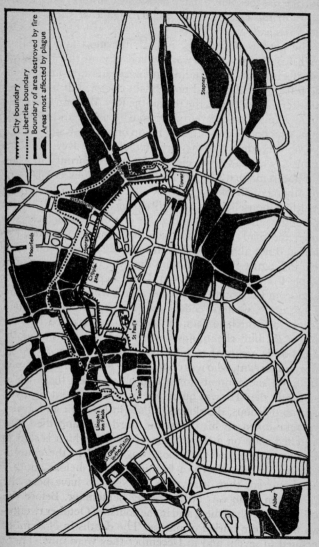

City boundary
Liberties boundary
Boundary of area destroyed by fire
Areas most affected by plague

Moorfields
Stepney
Tower
Cripple Gate
St Paul's
Temple
Lincoln's Inn Fields
St Clement Danes Fields
Abbey

4. Map of London showing areas affected by the plague in 1665 and destroyed by fire in 1666

District has become a part of English history akin to the stories of the charge of the Light Brigade or the wreck of the *Birkenhead*.

The plague of Eyam is, indeed, the most famous of all English outbreaks. Eyam was a village of some three hundred and fifty inhabitants, standing among meadows around which the hills towered. It had no resident doctor, but it had two ministers. The one was the rector, the Rev. William Mompesson, a young man of twenty-seven, with a wife and two children, who had been settled in Eyam only a year and did not like it; the other was the former rector, the Rev. Thomas Stanley, who had been ejected for nonconformity in 1662 and had remained to carry on his ministrations as a Dissenter among such of his old flock as adhered to him. The wealthier householders resided at the western and higher end of the village, on the other side of a brook which crossed under the road; as we shall see, they escaped the infection almost, if not altogether. The annual village wake had been held in August 1665 with more than the usual concourse of people from villages near. On 2 or 3 September a box arrived from London to the village tailor, who lived in a small house at the western end of the churchyard; it contained old clothes which someone in London is supposed to have bought for him cheap, and some tailors' patterns of cloth. This box is assumed to have been opened by one George Vicars, a servant, who was certainly the first victim of plague. He found the contents to be damp and hung them up at the fire to dry. He was quickly seized with violent sickness, became delirious, developed buboes in his neck and groin, a plague-token on his breast the third day, and died in a wretched state on 2 September. His body, which is said to have become putrid very soon, was buried in the churchyard on the 7th. Nearly a fortnight passed before another case occurred, that of a youth supposed to have been the tailor's son, who was buried on 22 September. Before the 30th four more had died, and in the course of October twenty-two more were buried of plague. The deaths in November declined to seven, and in December they were nine. There was now snow on the ground, with hard frost, and at the beginning of January 1666 the plague was confined to two houses. Four died in January, eight in February, six in March, nine in April, and only three in May. On 2 June another burial occurred, and then there was another pause. But in a week or more the epidemic broke out with renewed power, three having been buried on the 12th June, three on the 15th, one on the 16th, three on the 17th, and so on until the total for June reached nineteen. The wealthier villagers at the west end had taken the alarm before and had mostly fled in the spring; those who stayed kept within their houses or at least did not cross the stream. Now that the infection was revived in the hot weather of June, the rector's wife also proposed flight, but on her husband's refusal she resolved to remain with him, and to send her two children to a relative in Yorkshire. At the same time the villagers in general were instinctively moved to escape from the tainted spot; but Mompesson used his authority to prevent them, and a boundary line was drawn round the village, about half a mile in circuit and marked by various familiar objects, beyond which no one was to go. Mompesson's motive appears to have been to prevent the spread of the infection to the country around, and his parishioners submitted passively. After the end of June the villagers would have found it difficult to escape, owing to the terror which the very name of their village caused in all the country round. Some of them quitted their cottages and took up their abode in shelters built along the side of a rocky glen within the cordon. The Earl of Devonshire, then at Chatsworth, promised Mompesson that the village should not be left without supplies; and people from the villages near brought their market produce to certain stated points on the boundary, where the Eyam people came to fetch it, the money paid being dropped into water. Thus shut up in their narrow valley, the villagers perished helplessly like a stricken flock of sheep. By the end of June ceremonial burials came to an end, the church and the churchyard were closed, the dead were carried out wrapped in sheets by one of the villagers noted for his herculean strength, and laid in shallow graves in the meadows or on the hillsides. In July the deaths mounted up to five or six on some days, and the total for the month to fifty-seven. In August the dead numbered seventy-eight, among them the rector's wife, on the 25th, after a walk with her husband through the meadows, during which she is said to have made the ominous remark that the air smelled sweet! September added twenty-four to the total, and there were now only about forty-five left alive in the place. Of these, fifteen died up to 11 October, when the mortality ceased. Some of the survivors had passed through an attack of the plague, among them the rector's man, whose buboes suppurated. Mompesson himself, who had an issue open in his leg all the time, escaped the infection, as well as his maid-servant.

When the sickness had ceased Mompesson set about burning the infected articles in the empty cottages. Three years after, in 1669, he was presented to the better living of Eakring, in Notts; but on arriving to enter on his duties he was refused admission by the villagers, and had to take up his residence in a temporary hut in Rufford Park, until such time as the prejudices of his new parishioners had been overcome. Between September 1665 and October 1666, 259 inhabitants died of plague at Eyam and only thirty-three were left alive. Mompesson's action has often been criticized; yet although the cost was terrible, his action certainly saved the surrounding villages from plague.

Creighton* writes the obituary of plague in Britain in the following words:

Plague had been the grand infective disease of Britain from the year of the Black Death 1348-9 for more than three centuries, down to 1666. The last of plague in Scotland was in 1647-8, in the west and north-west of England about 1650, in Wales probably in 1636-8, in Ireland in 1650, and in all other parts of the kingdom in 1666, the absolute last of its provincial prevalence having been at Peterborough in the first months of 1667, while two or three deaths continued to occur annually in London down to 1679.

There is an interesting but undramatic postscript to that obituary, but first it is desirable to say something of the

---

* Creighton, 1894.

various theories which have been put forward to explain the disappearance of plague from England.

Perhaps the first, chronologically, is that the Great Fire of 1666 destroyed the seeds of infection so thoroughly that the disease never appeared again. Defoe* ascribed this theory to certain 'quacking' philosophers. There is a modern variant of this suggestion, put forward after the discovery of the mechanism of infection, which postulates that after the fire there was much rebuilding in brick and stone where wood and plaster had been before, and that the new brick and stone houses offered a much less favourable breeding ground for rats than did the old. The insuperable objection to the theory is that it is too parochial. Even if we confine our viewpoint to London we find that the area destroyed by fire was a mere fraction of the whole (Figure 4) and was the part least affected by plague. Plague began and throve not in the comparatively prosperous City but in the rat-ridden, wooden hovels of the poor in the Liberties and Out-parishes. These were hardly touched by the fire of 1666. If we survey the story of plague in western Europe as a whole we find that, except for a serious outbreak in Marseille and Provence in 1720-2, it had disappeared everywhere by about 1700.

Creighton† himself suggested that the disappearance of plague was due to a great increase in the use of coffins for burial which prevented the contamination of the soil by plague-infected bodies. This idea, like many of Creighton's explanations as opposed to his purely historical writing, seems to have been peculiar to himself. It need not, perhaps, be taken very seriously.

A theory put forward in many books, notably in Trevelyan's great *Social History*,‡ is that plague disappeared because the brown rat displaced the black. The black rat is more domesticated than the brown and is a better climber. At the present day it is found in ships and in high buildings, particularly in ports, but elsewhere it has been wholly replaced by the brown rat. Both types of rat are susceptible to plague, and both harbour fleas which will attack man when their normal

* D. Defoe, 1722.   † C. Creighton, 1894.
‡ G. M. Trevelyan, 1942.

37

host is dead. Thus this theory depends essentially on the difference in the social habits of the two species – the black rat lives closer to man than does the brown.

The great difficulty about accepting the rat theory is that of chronology. Plague, to all intents and purposes, disappeared from England in 1666 and from the whole of western Europe at about the same time with the single exception of the epidemic in the south of France about 1720. The earliest date given for the arrival of the brown rat in England, 1688, is a legendary one, for the rat is said to have arrived in the ship which brought William III from Holland. In fact the brown rat probably arrived considerably later – in 1728 or 1729 according to Pennant.* As late as 1783 Swaine, a rat catcher (quoted by Barrett-Hamilton and Hinton†), said that the black rat was the common one in London, Middlesex, and Buckinghamshire, but that elsewhere in the Home Counties the brown had ousted it. It would be reasonable to expect a long interval of freedom from plague in London after the great outburst of 1665–6, but to fit the rat theory, one must postulate an interval of a hundred years.

Other theories of the disappearance of plague are more vague. Liston‡ in his Milroy Lectures put forward the idea that epidemic diseases are a reflection of states of civilization. He pointed out that many of the diseases which we now regard as tropical diseases, for example, plague and malaria, were once serious problems in Britain. He ascribed the disappearance of plague to a gradual rise in the state of civilization. It is difficult to prove or disprove this theory, but it is doubtful whether the general state of civilization of the poor in large cities, particularly in London, was much higher in 1765 than in 1665. The deaths from other diseases of poverty, for example typhus, rose rather than fell, and this was the age of cheap gin drawn so vividly by Hogarth in 'Gin Lane'.

The conclusion must be that we do not really know why plague disappeared so suddenly when it did, and it remains

* T. Pennant, 1776–7.
† G. E. H. Barrett-Hamilton and M. A. C. Hinton, 1910–21.
‡ W. Glen Liston, 1924.

38

for us to consider events which are comparatively recent history and probably associated with the pandemic of plague which first became apparent at Hong Kong in 1893-4 and, like the earlier pandemics, spread over most of the inhabited world though with different results from those of its predecessors.

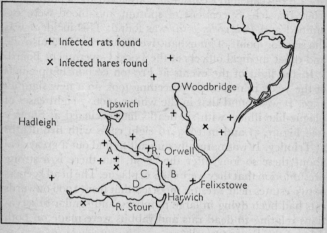

5. *Plague in East Anglia, 1906–18.*

A: *Freston, 4 confirmed cases 1910 (all died)*
B: *Trimley, 8 suspected cases 1909–10 (5 died)*
C: *Shotley, 8 suspected cases 1906–7 (6 died)*
   1 confirmed case 1911 (died)
D: *Erwarton, 2 confirmed cases 1918 (both died)*

So far as is known, plague never occurred in Britain between the late seventeenth century and the beginning of the twentieth. In 1900 and 1901 there were a few cases in Glasgow, and in 1901 probably eleven in Liverpool and one in Cardiff. All these occurred in large ports, and although it was not always possible to trace the source of infection it seems reasonable to suppose that they were directly associated with rats from ships.

An incident which occurred in 1910 is of more interest in that it implied a much deeper and more lasting penetration of infection. In the winter of 1910–11 there occurred four cases of an extremely virulent type of pneumonia in the little village of Freston (see Figure 5). Three of these cases were in one family, and the fourth was that of a neighbour who had nursed the mother during her illness. All four patients died. The family doctor was puzzled by the virulence of the disease and called in a consultant physician and a pathologist from Ipswich. Specimens of sputum and blood were examined and *Pasteurella pestis* was found. This incident was the starting-point of an exhaustive inquiry by Dr Bulstrode and other medical officers of the Local Government Board.

In the light of the events at Freston certain happenings of the years immediately preceding took on a new significance. It was found that in the winter 1906–7 eight cases of plague-like illness with six deaths had occurred at Shotley (see Figure 5) and in 1909–10 eight cases with five deaths at Trimley. It was naturally difficult to find out a great deal about these so long after the event, but there is a strong presumption that they were cases of plague. The head keepers of two estates near Freston reported that from 1906 onwards rats had been dying in large numbers, and similar observations relating to dead rats and rabbits were made on both sides of the River Orwell.

After the cases at Freston a widespread search was made for infected rodents, and the results of the search are indicated on the map. The search was kept up for several years, and infected rodents were occasionally found even as late as 1918. There were three more cases of human plague in the district, one in a seaman at Shotley naval barracks in 1911 and two at Erwarton (see Figure 5). Nearly all the human cases occurred in poor homes with an abundance of fleas.

There seems to be little doubt therefore that rodent plague was well established in this part of Suffolk from 1906 to 1918, and yet only twenty-three human cases were reported in the whole period. There can be little doubt that the spread of plague is very unlikely in a community with standards of living similar to those in an English rural district. There is other evidence for this belief, for plague is now established in the wild rodent populations of no fewer than fifteen of the

Western States of the United States; there were, for example, six human cases in New Mexico in 1949, but there has never been a larger scale epidemic.

Although, for the reasons already given, we cannot ascribe the disappearance of plague from western Europe to a rising standard of civilization, it does seem reasonable to attribute its recent failure to spread to the changes in standards of living since the seventeenth century.

3

INFLUENZA – THE SWEATING SICKNESS

INFLUENZA is caused by a virus first described by Wilson Smith, Andrewes, and Laidlow* in 1933.

The demonstration of the existence of the influenza virus by the British workers mentioned above opened a new chapter in the study of the disease, and since then an immense amount of work has been done. This work on viruses is highly technical and complex, and any brief description must necessarily be an over-simplification. Briefly there are two important influenza viruses, A and B. Virus A is the one usually found in major epidemics, whereas B tends to occur in more localized outbreaks – in camps, schools, and the like. The virus discovered in 1933 was A, but since then many other strains of A which differ from the original and from each other have been isolated. There is a general belief among those who work with influenza viruses that a succession of changes is occurring in them. Strains of A isolated in different parts of the world at about the same time tend to resemble one another more than those isolated a few years earlier. Even in non-epidemic years some deaths are attributed to influenza but in such years a virus can rarely be isolated. In order to explain this Andrewes has suggested that there may be a 'basic' influenza virus which is not detectable by the laboratory tests at present available but which can cause illness and occasionally death. In an epidemic year, this virus becomes changed in some way, acquires the power of spread, and can be detected by laboratory tests.

It is relatively easy to write about plague because the clinical features of the disease are sufficiently characteristic to enable one to identify epidemics far back into antiquity. With influenza the position is very different. All that one can do is to search the records for examples of epidemics,

* W. Smith, C. H. Andrewes, and P. P. Laidlow, 1933.

or preferably pandemics, of a disease with symptoms mainly connected with the respiratory tract, with an acute onset, a very high attack rate, and, on the whole, a low case mortality. Some of these characteristics are very variable. For example, in some epidemics the respiratory symptoms may be very obvious whilst in others they may be almost absent. In some, notably that of 1918–19, the total mortality has been enormous, though even in that pandemic it must be remembered that the number of cases far exceeded the number of deaths. In some communities in 1918–19 almost every member was attacked, so that the pandemic did satisfy the criterion of a relatively low case fatality.

From the historical point of view the discovery of the virus of influenza by Wilson Smith, Andrewes, and Laidlow in 1933 is recent and does not help in the identification of the epidemics of the past. For the identification of these we have to rely on a blend of clinical and epidemiological description and must often be in doubt as to whether the disease was or was not influenza. Some descriptions are, however, extremely lifelike and it may be permissible to quote a particularly good one out of its strict chronological order. This was written by Willis* and relates to an epidemic in 1658:

About the end of April, suddenly a Distemper arose, as if sent by some blast of the stars, which laid hold on very many together: that in some towns, in the space of a week, above a thousand people fell sick together. The particular symptom of this disease, and which first invaded the sick, was a troublesome cough, with great spitting, also a catarrh fallin down on the palat, throat, and nostrils; also it was accompanied with a feaverish distemper, joyned with heat and thirst, want of appetite, a spontaneous weariness, and a grievous pain in the back and limbs: which feaver, however, was more remiss in some, that they could go abroad, and follow their affairs in the time of their sickness, but complaining, in the mean time of want of strength and of languishing, a loathing of food, a cough, and a catarrh. But in some a very hot distemper plainly appeared, that being thrown into bed they were troubled with burning thirst, waking hoarseness, and coughing almost continual: sometimes there came upon this a bleeding at the nose, and in some a bloody spittle, and frequently a bloody flux; such as were indued with an infirm

* T. Willis, 1659.

body, or men of a more declining age, that were taken with this disease, not a few died of it; but the more strong, and almost all of an healthful constitution, recovered: those who falling sick of this disease and died, for the most part died by reason of the strength being leisurely wasted, and a serous heap more and more gathered together in the breast, with the feaver being increased, and a difficulty of breath, like those sick of an hectic feaver. Concerning this disease, we are to enquire, what procatartic cause it had, that it should arise in the middle of the Spring suddenly, and that the third part of makind, almost, should be distempered with the same, in the space of a month: then the signs and symptoms being carefully collated, the formal reason of this disease, also its crisis and way of cure, ought to be assigned.

Anyone reading that description today must feel convinced that Willis saw an epidemic of influenza.

According to Thompson* the first identifiable epidemic of influenza in England was in 1510. The clinical description is similar to that of Willis already quoted, but is shorter. Something is said of its origin, in Malta, and of its spread. The epidemic spread rapidly and involved the whole of Europe. According to Creighton† there is no contemporary evidence of this epidemic in English writings, but certain foreign writers stated that England was affected.

One of the most intriguing epidemiological problems of these early years is that of the identity of the disease known as the Sweating Sickness or English Sweat. Was it influenza or was it not? The main facts about it as given by Creighton† are as follows: It appeared suddenly in 1485 either just before or soon after the battle of Bosworth (22 August 1485). It was raging in London at the end of September and in October, and two mayors and four aldermen died of it. There is no very detailed account of the clinical course of the disease in this epidemic, but it seems to have been rapidly fatal – sometimes within six hours of onset. The sweating from which the disease took its name was a prominent symptom. The best known description of the disease is that of John Caius‡ and relates to the last epidemic – that of 1551. Between 1485 and 1551, there were five epidemics, in 1485, 1508, 1517,

* T. Thompson, 1820.　　　　† C. Creighton, 1894.
‡ John Caius, 1552.

1528, and 1551, and then all references to the disease ceased so far as England was concerned. Creighton* quotes many contemporary references to the Sweating Sickness and it seems to be reasonably well established that the disease usually occurred in the summer and autumn, attacking the rich rather than the poor, often having a high mortality rate among young adults, and killing very quickly. There seems to be no mention of respiratory symptoms in the contemporary accounts. It is hard to recognize similarities between these contemporary descriptions and influenza as we know it, and the only disease of modern times which seems to have a likeness to the English Sweat is the disease described in France and known as the Picardy Sweat. There is an interesting short article on Sweating Sickness by Michael Foster† in the memorial volume dedicated to Osler on the occasion of his seventieth birthday. Foster was inspired to investigate the subject because he had seen a case of Picardy Sweat while serving in France in the First World War. He points out that there is a marked similarity between the symptoms described by Caius – profuse sweating, palpitation, epigastric pain, and fear of imminent death – and those described by the French writers on the Picardy Sweat. The chief difference between the clinical descriptions is that the French writers describe a miliary rash which is not mentioned in the Tudor records. There seems to be little doubt that the Picardy Sweat is not the same disease as influenza, but whether it is the same disease as the English Sweat is more doubtful. On the whole the clinical evidence is against the identification of either the English Sweat or the Picardy Sweat with influenza. The relatively short space of time (1485–1551) during which epidemics of the English Sweat were occurring is roughly the same as that in which epidemics of respiratory diseases began to be reported following the pandemic of what was probably influenza in 1510 which has already been mentioned. There were epidemics of acute respiratory diseases which spread over Europe in 1580–2.

In the first half of the seventeenth century there were few such outbreaks, but in 1658 occurred the epidemic described

* C. Creighton, 1894.   † M.G. Foster, 1919.

by Willis in the passage quoted earlier in this chapter. From 1661 to 1686 Sydenham* was writing his account of the seasons and reigning diseases of London and he makes many references to outbreaks of respiratory disease which may or may not have been epidemics of influenza. As has been said in the previous chapter, Sydenham's field of vision was somewhat limited, as he was a fashionable physician practising in London and so did not know much of what was happening elsewhere in the country or even perhaps in the poorer parts of London itself. One observation of Sydenham's has been of particular interest to epidemiologists of a later age; this refers to the epidemic of 1685 in which Sydenham says that symptoms of disease of the nervous system were particularly prevalent. It is not easy to decide what disease Sydenham was describing, but it may have been meningococcal meningitis or possibly encephalitis lethargica.

The chief difficulty in interpreting the writings of the great clinicians of the Restoration is in deciding how widespread were the epidemics which they described, and it is in fact extremely difficult to make any estimate of the scale of epidemics until much later, when national statistics began in 1837. Some attempt seems to have been made to estimate the extent of an epidemic of influenza in 1782, when the Royal College of Physicians by public advertisement asked for information from the physicians of Great Britain about the extent of the epidemic of influenza then occurring. They collected information from all over the country and were able to establish that the disease started at Newcastle at the end of April 1782 and appeared in London between 12 and 18 May and in the Eastern Counties about the middle of May. This seems to have been the first attempt to collect information on a national scale. Throughout the eighteenth and early nineteenth centuries there were many outbreaks of influenza, but it is not possible to determine whether these were pandemic on the scale of those which occurred later. There is little doubt that in 1837–41 there was a widespread prevalence of influenza in Europe, and England was certainly affected. These were the early years of the General Register

* T. Sydenham, 1676.

46

Office and, although the collection of information about deaths by cause was then very imperfect, it is perhaps worth mentioning that, in the year 1841, 1,659 deaths from influenza were registered and 220 of these occurred in London. The next explosion was in 1847–8, and in those two years some 15,000 deaths were ascribed to this cause. From then to 1861 the deaths registered every year exceeded 1,000, but from 1861 to 1889 they were insignificant, and Greenwood* in his summary of the history of influenza in the Ministry of Health report on the epidemic of 1918 says, 'In 1889 this country had been free from pandemic influenza for more years than in any previous epoch since the middle of the seventeenth century'.

The pandemic of 1889–92 was the beginning of a new chapter in the history of the disease not only in England and Wales but also in Europe and North America and probably throughout the world. Since 1889 influenza has been an appreciable cause of death in many years both before and after the greatest pandemic of all time – that of 1918–19.

There are conflicting statements as to the origin of the pandemic of 1889–92 but it seems to be established that Russia was affected in the early winter of 1889. Clemow† writing in the *Lancet* of 1894 produces reasonably convincing evidence of spread from western Siberia at the end of September to European Russia, but the spread was extremely rapid and the disease appeared in St Petersburg (now Leningrad) in October. By the end of December, most of continental Europe was affected, and by the middle of December influenza was reported in New York and Boston. A few cases began to be reported in London early in December, but the epidemic reached its height there about 11 January and was declining rapidly by 8 February.

A problem which is always discussed during a pandemic of influenza is whether the epidemic begins in one country and spreads to others, or whether it begins in several centres at about the same time. In 1889–90 the disease was known in western Europe as 'Russian influenza', but whether the pandemic really had its origin there must be regarded as

* L. H. Greenwood.   † D. Clemow, 1894.

still unsettled. In his comments on this point, the Medical Officer of the Local Government Board (*Ann. Rept. 1889–90*) was clearly sceptical on this question of naming any particular country as the country of origin.

The behaviour of the disease after 1889–90 resembled that after the pandemic of 1918–19 in that there were recurrent

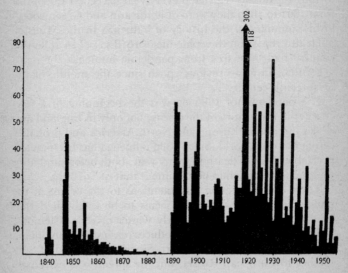

6. *Deaths from influenza in England and Wales per 100,000 of population, 1840–1955*

waves of disease in the years following. These are shown in Figure 6 from which it will be seen that the death rate fell irregularly but remained at a higher level than before right up to the pandemic of 1918.

In spite of the fact that there is no exact information from many countries about numbers of cases or even of deaths there can be little doubt that the total number of cases in the pandemic of influenza of 1918–19 was the greatest outbreak of pestilence that the human race has ever experienced. It is too recent an event to be seen in full historical perspective, and perhaps some historian of the future will be able to see that it had effects on world history comparable with those of the Justinian Plague or the Black Death. More probably, however, it may never have an important place in the history books because the vast majority of those who had the disease had a relatively short illness, even though it was very unpleasant while it lasted. The number of deaths in England and Wales directly attributable to influenza was approximately 150,000. No one knows how many died in the whole world, but a rough guess of 15 millions has been made. Like the disease itself, the pandemic was short and sharp. It began in the early summer of 1918 and reached its climax in the autumn and winter of 1918–19. A unique feature of this pandemic was that all over the world it tended to kill the young and vigorous rather than the old and weak. The report of the Ministry of Health has a section of 200 pages devoted to reports from nearly every country in the world, and in the whole of that record there are only two places – the islands of St Helena and the South Pacific – which are reported to have escaped.

In England and Wales it was possible to distinguish three waves of prevalence. The first was in June–July 1918, and though the attack rate was high the disease was, on the whole, not severe. The second was in October and November 1918 and in this the disease was much more severe and tended to kill the young rather than the elderly. It was at this time that most of the fatal cases with heliotrope cyanosis occurred. The third wave, in February 1919 was also severe, but less so than the second, and the mortality in the young was less marked.

After the pandemic of 1918–19 there was a period of about ten years during which the annual death rates tended to remain high both in epidemic and in non-epidemic years, but since 1929 the tendency has been downward both in epidemic and in non-epidemic years. The concentration of mortality on those aged 15–35, which was so new a feature of the pandemic period, did not persist for more than two or three years, and soon there was a complete reversion to the kind of disease which was relatively trivial for the young.

No one can prophesy what the future of influenza will

be, but the temptation to speculate a little is irresistible. Is it likely that a pandemic on the scale of that of 1918–19 may occur again, and if so will the new drugs which have been discovered since then be so effective that the death rate will be negligible, at any rate among those in youth and early middle age? It seems probable that there will be pandemics in the future as there have been in the past and, although we shall be able to learn much more about them now that we can study the causative virus, it is unlikely that we shall be able to do a great deal to prevent their spread. It may be possible to prepare effective vaccines, but it will not be easy to prepare them quickly enough and on a sufficiently large scale to protect whole populations.

It is more difficult to make even a guess at the probable effectiveness of the new drugs, such as penicillin. Probably none of those known at present is effective against the influenza virus itself, but we do not know whether it was the influenza virus which killed so many people in the prime of life in 1918–19 or whether the worst damage was done by secondary bacterial invaders. The omens are favourable if secondary infection did the damage and less favourable if the virus itself did. There is one small piece of statistical evidence recently put forward by Logan* which gives ground for a little optimism. He showed that in the most recent outbreak of 1951, the proportion of the total number of deaths among persons over fifty-five was no less than 88 per cent – higher than in 1933 (59 per cent) and far higher than in 1918 (14 per cent). All this is, however, pure speculation, and all that the epidemiologist can do is to keep a weather eye open for the danger signals which heralded the pandemic of 1918 – an outbreak in the summer with a sudden age shift of mortality from old people to younger ones.

* W.P.D.Logan, see W.H.Bradley, 1951.

4

LEPROSY – THE GREAT POX
(SYPHILIS) – SMALLPOX

To the modern reader leprosy, syphilis, and smallpox may seem to have little in common, but in medieval times there was much confusion between diseases in which unpleasant lesions of the skin were found, and the term leprosy in particular was probably used to describe a multitude of skin conditions. Leprosy is caused by a bacillus which, under the microscope, looks like the tubercle bacillus. The bacillus was discovered by Hansen* in 1871. Contrary to popular belief, leprosy is not readily communicated from one person to another, and those who contract the disease are people who have lived with lepers for many years. The only reason for mentioning it in this book is the possible confusion with syphilis in medieval times. Syphilis is caused by a spiral organism discovered by Schaudinn in 1905, and is communicated by intimate contact, nearly always by sexual intercourse. Smallpox is caused by a virus which is large as viruses go, having a diameter of about 300 mμ. Smallpox is one of the most infectious diseases known, and it has even been suspected that the virus could be carried by the wind from a smallpox hospital, to infect persons at a considerable distance from the building.

LEPROSY AND SYPHILIS

It may be well to consider leprosy first, as there is little to be said about it and, from the chronological point of view, the disease was important only at the beginning of the period covered by this book. Creighton† considers that true leprosy undoubtedly existed in England in medieval times. He quotes a description by Gilbertus Anglicus of which the date is unknown in which the following characteristic signs and symptoms are described: ' The eyebrows falling bare and getting

* G. H. A. Hansen, 1874.   † C. Creighton, 1894.

knotted with uneven tuberosities, the nose and other features becoming thick, coarse, and lumpy, the face losing its mobility or play of expression, the raucous voice, the loss of sensibility in the hands, and the ultimate break-up or maufragium of the leprous growths into foul running sores'. It seems likely that true leprosy was declining at the end of the fourteenth century and had disappeared by the fifteenth. The great interest of Creighton's chapter on the subject lies rather in the references to skin conditions which were almost certainly not leprosy at all and which may have been syphilis. Creighton quotes a whole series of references from the beginning of the fourteenth century onwards to the venereal origin of leprosy and mentions an edict of Edward III to the mayor and sheriffs of London in 1346 instructing them to drive out lepers from the City. One of the main reasons given is that lepers 'communicate their disease by carnal intercourse with women in stews and other secret places'. Some of the clinical descriptions given sound remarkably like the lesions of secondary syphilis.

Whatever the lesions of the skin which were called leprosy really were, there is no doubt that, in the last years of the fifteenth century there was an extraordinary pandemic of syphilis in Europe. If it were not for this, syphilis could have had no place in this book, for since then it has been an endemic and not an epidemic disease. Many thousands of words have been written by medical historians about the origin of this pandemic of syphilis. The controversy began early in the sixteenth century and is still unsettled. One school believes passionately that syphilis was brought back from America by sailors who accompanied Columbus on his second voyage, and their story runs roughly as follows: Columbus left Seville on 4 August 1492, landed on Haiti, and returned to Palos, 500 miles from Barcelona, on 15 March 1493. Many of the forty-four who returned with Columbus were infected with syphilis and very soon after their return an epidemic of an extremely acute and fatal form of the disease broke out in Barcelona. In 1494 Charles VIII of France was preparing for an invasion of Italy and in his army was a body of Spanish mercenaries under Gonzalo de

Cordoba. At about the time of the occupation of Naples from February to May 1495 the disease became widely disseminated in the army and in Italy generally, and from there it spread all over Europe, reaching Scotland by 1497 and London at least as early as 1503.*

The other school believes just as passionately that syphilis had occurred in Europe from time immemorial but that, up to the end of the fifteenth and beginning of the sixteenth centuries, it had been a less acute and fatal illness and had been confused with leprosy and many other skin diseases. For some unknown reason there was at this time a pandemic of an extremely acute and fatal form of the disease which probably began in France and Spain and spread rapidly over the whole of Europe. The change of type lasted some twenty or thirty years, and then the disease reverted to the more chronic form of today.

The first original English writer on the Morbus Gallicus, or Morbus Neapolitanus as he called it, was William Clowes, who published his treatise in 1579. He was surgeon to St Bartholomew's Hospital and had treated many cases with inunctions of mercury. His descriptions suggest that the disease had by then lost the terrible severity of the original epidemic type.

The origin of the European pandemic remains a mystery and, quite apart from the controversy over historical details, the alternative explanations both present serious difficulties to the epidemiologist. On the one hand it is difficult to believe that the disease could have travelled so far and so fast from a single place and, on the other, it is difficult to explain the sudden change of type if one accepts the view that syphilis had been endemic in Europe for centuries.

SMALLPOX

As epidemic diseases, leprosy and syphilis disappeared from the scene long ago, but smallpox had a long innings, and we have not seen the last of it even now. The early history of smallpox in England is obscure. In the medieval period

* C. Creighton, I (1894), p. 419.

there are scattered references to 'pockes', but it is not certain whether these refer to syphilis, smallpox, or possibly even to other skin diseases. For some mysterious reason the champions of vaccination of a later age seem to have felt that it was necessary to their argument to show that smallpox was a common and deadly disease in the Middle Ages, whereas the opponents of vaccination tended to attribute these references to other diseases and to consider that smallpox was a new disease in the England of the Tudors. Whatever one may think of Creighton's views on the value of vaccination, one cannot help respecting him as a historian, and his general account of the history of smallpox carries more conviction than does that of his opponents. It is difficult to improve on Creighton's own summary:

The history of smallpox in Britain is that of a disease coming gradually into prominence and hardly attaining a leading place until the reign of James I. In this respect it is unlike plague and sweating sickness, both of which burst upon the country in their full strength, just as both made their last show in epidemics which were as severe as any in their history.

In a later passage he says:

It would be a not incorrect summary of the incidence of smallpox in Britain to say that it first left the richer classes, then it left the villages, then it left the provincial towns, to centre itself in the capital; at the same time it was leaving the age of infancy and childhood. Of course it did none of these things absolutely but the movement in any one of those directions has been as obvious as in any other. Measles and scarlatina have not shown the same tendency to change or limit their incidence. Smallpox may have surprises in store for us; but, as an exotic infection, its peculiar behaviour may not unreasonably be taken to mean that it is dying out – dying as in the death of some individuals, gradually from the extremities to the heart.

That was written in 1894 and Creighton was convinced that vaccination was ineffective in preventing smallpox. His argument that the chief determining factor in the history of smallpox has been the natural history of the disease itself, unaffected by vaccination, is one for which there is much to be said, but in the following pages we shall have to consider the other side of the argument and also to describe some of the surprises which smallpox had in store in 1894.

The number of deaths recorded each year in the London Bills from 1729 to the beginning of death registration (1837) is shown in Figure 7a. These can, of course, be regarded

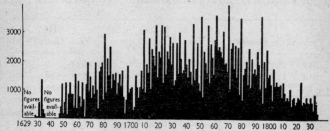

7 (a). *Deaths from smallpox in London, 1629–1837. Compiled from the Bills of Mortality*

only as a very rough guide to the actual number of deaths, and it must also be remembered that over this long period London was growing enormously and that the movement of population from the City into the surrounding Liberties and Out-parishes was beginning. From time to time the area covered by the Bills was extended but St Pancras, St Marylebone, Chelsea, and Kensington were never included in them. The Bills are a particularly inaccurate guide at the end of the period and there is a very marked discrepancy between the figure given in them for the year 1837 – 217 – and the number of deaths actually registered in the period 1 July–31 December 1837 – 762. In spite of the inaccuracies of the Bills, Creighton considers that they may be taken as showing, on the whole fairly, the proportion of deaths from smallpox to those from other causes and the years of its greatest outbursts. Figure 7b shows the annual death rates in England and Wales from smallpox from the first full year of registration (1838) to 1905. The epidemic of 1900–5 was the last considerable outbreak of major smallpox in Britain, and after it the annual death rates reached a very low figure. The end of major smallpox as a 'native' disease was less sudden than that of plague, but it is probably true to say that since the time of the First World War major smallpox has been exotic. It is impossible to prove this thesis because it has not always been possible to trace the source of the many small outbreaks, but it seems plausible.

The trend of smallpox from 1911 to 1955 is shown in the table below of notifications and deaths recorded in each year.

I				II			III		
Year	Cases	Deaths		Year	Cases	Deaths	Year	Cases	Deaths
1911	295	23		1923	2485	7	1935	1	–
1912	123	9		1924	3765	13	1936	12	–
1913	115	10		1925	5365	9	1937	3	–
1914	64	4	Minor Smallpox	1926	10146	18	1938	18	–
1915	90	13		1927	14767	47	1939	1	–
1916	149	16		1928	12420	53	1940	1	–
1917	7	3		1929	10967	39	1941	–	–
1918	63	2		1930	11839	28	1942	7	–
1919	294	24		1931	5664	9	1943	–	–
1920	263	30		1932	2039	3	1944	16	3
1921	315	5		1933	631	2	1945	4	–
1922	973	27		1934	179	6	1946	56	14
							1947	78	15
							1948	–	–
							1949	19	5
							1950	8	–
							1951	27	10
							1952	135	1
							1953	30	8
							1954	–	–
							1955	–	–

If one compares the three columns of this table it is immediately obvious that smallpox had indeed one great surprise in store when Creighton wrote of it as a dying disease in 1894. In the summer of 1919 there was a small outbreak of smallpox in Norfolk and Suffolk in which the disease had quite different clinical characteristics from those usually associated with smallpox. It was far milder than that experienced in former years and was very rarely fatal. In 1920 there was another outbreak of this minor smallpox in Lancashire with 83 known cases and not a single death. Throughout

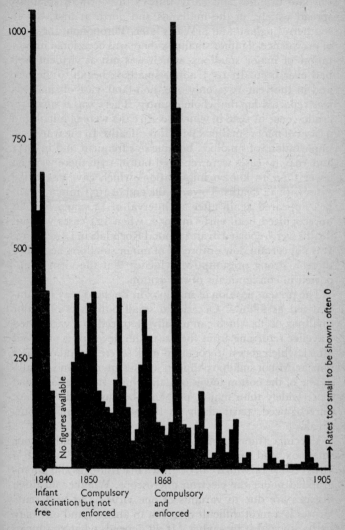

7 (b). *Deaths from smallpox in England and Wales in the period from the beginning of registration to 1905*

the late twenties and early thirties this form of smallpox spread widely, in the midlands and north at first, but in southern England and in Wales later. Throughout the years of prevalence of minor smallpox there was occasional importation of major smallpox, which was just as virulent as it had ever been. In 1931 minor smallpox began to die out, and in the year 1935 only one, non-fatal, case of smallpox was reported for the whole country. There was a small recrudescence in 1938 in which year 9 cases were of minor and 9 cases of major smallpox with three deaths. In the war years importations of smallpox became less frequent and in 1941 and 1943 no cases were reported but in 1946 there were no fewer than 15 known importations which gave rise to 56 cases with 14 deaths. Towards the end of 1951 minor smallpox appeared again after an interval of 13 years. It went unrecognized until early in 1952, when 124 cases without deaths were reported in and around Rochdale in Lancashire. It is not certain how outbreaks of minor smallpox begin but there is strong presumptive evidence that the virus is imported in consignments of raw cotton.

The present position of smallpox in England may be summarized as follows. Occasional small outbreaks of major smallpox occur which can usually be traced to a vaccinated traveller returning from the East who develops a modified attack which goes unrecognized until severe secondary cases appear. Minor smallpox appears at long intervals and usually in one of the cotton towns of Lancashire. It tends to spread more widely than major, probably because mild cases are unrecognized, particularly in the early stages of an outbreak.

Vaccinia (the lesions produced by vaccination), minor smallpox, and major smallpox are due to infection with a virus or viruses, which can be grown in fertile eggs and photographed under the electron microscope. Whether all three diseases are due to variants of one virus or to 'different' viruses is a most difficult question to answer, and one may perhaps avoid it by saying, 'It all depends what you mean by different', and by summarizing the likenesses and differences. In the laboratory, material obtained from all three diseases behaves in much the same way, though there are slight differences between the appearances produced in the fertile egg by material from vaccinia and those produced by material from major or minor smallpox. An attack of one disease produces strong immunity against the other two. As human diseases the three are very different. Vaccinia, as ordinarily produced by inoculation of glycerinated lymph, is nearly always a trivial affair of a small itching spot at the site of inoculation. Very rarely, however, the rash is generalized and the illness severe. Minor smallpox varies a good deal in severity but is, generally speaking, slightly more unpleasant than chicken-pox, whereas major smallpox is one of the most deadly infectious diseases known, with a mortality of the order of twenty-five per cent or more in the unvaccinated.

One of the most difficult tasks which confronts the historian of smallpox is to form a just estimate of the part played by inoculation and vaccination in contributing to the decline of the disease. The literature on the subject is enormous, and much has been written both by those who regard it as heresy to question for one moment the part played by vaccination and on the other hand by those who regard vaccination as an invention of the devil. It is important to distinguish between vaccination as a means of protecting an individual against smallpox and vaccination as a public health measure designed to protect a community against epidemics of the disease. There can be no doubt at all that vaccination repeated at intervals of five years or so will almost certainly protect an individual from smallpox. The problem is, however, to decide how far the limited amount of inoculation and vaccination which has been practised in England at different times has determined the trends of morbidity and mortality of the disease.

Inoculation with material derived from the pocks of patients suffering from mild attacks of smallpox had been practised from very early times. It was introduced into England about 1720, largely owing to the efforts of Lady Mary Wortley Montagu. Throughout the eighteenth century inoculation was practised with varying frequency and varying success.

Sometimes the patient had a mild attack and sometimes he had a severe or even fatal one. The procedure was, however, too chancy to become very popular, and with the introduction of vaccination in the early part of the nineteenth century it gradually fell into disuse. Inoculation was made a criminal offence in 1840.

In 1798 Edward Jenner published his famous *Inquiry into the Causes and Effects of the Variolae Vaccinae*. His argument rested on two propositions: (1) that those who had suffered from naturally acquired cowpox did not get smallpox, (2) that cowpox could be carried from arm to arm and would protect all those who had been cowpoxed against smallpox. In support of his first proposition he cited some twenty instances of persons who had had cowpox and had subsequently been given an inoculation of matter from a patient with smallpox without any ill-effect. The intervals between the attacks of cowpox and the test inoculations of smallpox varied from fifty-three years to nine months. In every case the test inoculation failed to produce smallpox. In support of his second proposition, Jenner cited his experiment of inoculating a child with matter from a dairymaid who had contracted natural cowpox and other children with matter from a cow suffering from the disease. He did not apply the test of smallpox inoculation to all these children but to only three of them. According to modern standards these experiments of Jenner's were rather thin, but they did arouse a great deal of attention in London, and in particular they stimulated Dr Woodville* of the Smallpox and Inoculation Hospital to undertake a clinical trial of the method. Dr Woodville's experiments are of particular interest as it seems possible that some of the vaccine lymph which is in use today may have had its ultimate ancestry in them. Unfortunately it is difficult to interpret the experiments. Woodville got his cowpox lymph from a cow in a dairy in Gray's Inn Lane, where 200 cows were kept of which some four-fifths were attacked. He inoculated seven persons with this material and subsequently inoculated these seven with smallpox matter at varying intervals. Three of them were inoculated after an interval of

* M. Woodville, 1799.

only five days. The subsequent history of Woodville's experiments is most confusing, because from the original seven he inoculated a whole series of other persons with matter from the local cowpox lesions and, at varying intervals afterwards, gave inoculations of material from cases of smallpox. In all he inoculated 200 persons in his first series and another 300 later. Some of them had generalized eruptions and a few were very ill. Anyone reading Woodville's own account now must be left with a strong suspicion that some of Woodville's patients had attacks of modified smallpox. He expressed his conclusions as follows:

Were I enabled to state a number of cases of variolous inoculation, equal to those given above, and reduced to a similar tabular form, the comparative magnitude of the two diseases might be estimated with tolerable precision. It is evident, however, that the matter of the vaccine disease has generally produced much fewer pustules, and less indisposition, than that of the smallpox; for it appears from the preceding statement that about two-fifths of all the persons inoculated for the Variolae Vaccinae had no pustules and that in not more than a fourth part of them was there experienced any perceptible disorder of the constitution. But it must be acknowledged that, in several instances, the cowpox has proved a very severe disease. In three or four cases out of five hundred, the patient has been in considerable danger, and one child, as I have already observed, actually died under the effects of the disease. Now, if it be admitted that, at an average, one of five hundred will die of the inoculated cowpox, I confess I should not be disposed to introduce this disease into the Inoculation Hospital, because out of the last five thousand cases of variolous inoculation the number of deaths has not exceeded the proportion of one in six hundred. But I am inclined to think that if the matter of the cowpox, used for the purpose of inoculation, were only taken from those in whom the disease appeared in a very mild form, the result would be more favourable than in the statement here given.

It is impossible to trace all the ramifications of the early history of vaccine lymph and it is difficult to interpret even so good an account of experiments as that of Woodville. One can only make a guess at what happened in London after 1799. The most plausible guess seems to me to be that the bringing together of cowpox and smallpox virus did in some way produce a modified smallpox virus which by an empirical process of selection (see Woodville's last sentence) on the part of the vaccinators gradually became safer and safer. The virus was kept going by arm to arm vaccination right up to 1881 when glycerinated calf lymph began to be substituted for it. Arm to arm vaccination was not finally prohibited till 1898. Modern work on viruses lends some support to this theory, in that, in the laboratory, the vaccinia virus resembles the smallpox virus rather more than the cowpox virus, though the cowpox virus has a similar antigenic structure.

Whatever may be the true origin of the vaccinia virus, it is reasonably certain that in the early years of the nineteenth century vaccination became recognized more and more as an effective method of preventing smallpox and even more as an effective method of preventing death from smallpox. The trend of deaths in London during the early years of the nineteenth century (see Figure 7a) suggests that some potent factor was at work which tended to diminish the number of deaths. It is true that there were substantial outbreaks of smallpox later in the century, particularly in 1871–2, and Greenwood* considered that the decline in the number of deaths in London was not a valid argument in favour of vaccination as a public health measure. Creighton also pointed out that the returns of the parish clerks in the early nineteenth century were particularly inaccurate. He forbore to point out, however, that the total number of deaths returned each year did not fall as did those from smallpox. The argument that vaccination had a good deal to do with the decline of deaths is, of course, an argument *post hoc ergo propter hoc*, but the alternative explanation that smallpox suddenly changed in type at just about the time vaccination was introduced seems more difficult to substantiate.

The year 1838 was the first full year of registration of deaths in England and Wales, and, with all their failings, the statistics available from that year onwards are incomparably more reliable and comprehensive than the earlier ones. The early years of registration correspond with the last

* L. H. Greenwood, 1935.

great epidemic 1837–40 which 'showed smallpox in its old colours' (Creighton). It is not possible to compare the numbers of deaths reported in this epidemic with those recorded in the Bills, because the area included in 'London' as a registration area was much larger than the area included in the Bills. There had also been great changes in population since the eighteenth century. It is, however, of some interest to note that the number of deaths from smallpox registered in London in 1838 (3,817) was only a little larger than the number (3,548) recorded in the Bills in 1796. This suggests a considerable reduction in mortality.

From 1840 to 1870 there was a fair amount of smallpox in England and Wales, but it was a mere shadow of its eighteenth-century self and began to change from a disease which killed children almost exclusively to one which caused deaths among older people also. In the eighteenth century some 80 per cent of the deaths were those of children under five, and nearly the whole of the remaining 20 per cent of children between five and ten; but in the registration period the age distribution changed, at first gradually, and then much more rapidly in the epidemic of 1871–2. In the period 1851–60 the deaths of children under five were 62 per cent of the total, in 1861–70 54 per cent, and in 1871–80 only 30 per cent. Another new characteristic of smallpox in the nineteenth century was its tendency to remain an important disease in London when it was dying out in the provinces:

Smallpox: *death-rates per million living*
(Creighton (1894), Vol. II, p. 617)

	1847–9	1850–4	1855–9	1860–4	1865–9	1870–4	1875–9	1880–4
London	460	300	237	281	276	654	292	244
Provinces	274	271	192	175	172	339	48	34

It is not possible to give exact estimates of the amount of vaccination carried out at any of these periods but information became more accurate throughout the second half of the century as the machinery of public health administration improved. Greenwood* considered that the amount of vaccination practised in London in the first twenty-five years

* L. H. Greenwood, I, p. 239.

of the nineteenth century was insignificant from the preventive point of view. No one knows how much vaccination was done, but Creighton* suggested that perhaps something like half the children born in London were vaccinated at this time. Clearly this was not enough to prevent epidemics, since that of 1837–40 was a severe one, but it seems reasonable to suppose that even in this period a good many lives were saved by vaccination. Infant vaccination was made available at the public expense in 1840 and compulsory in 1853, but the machinery of compulsion was inefficient, and it was not until 1868 that steps were taken to enforce the vaccination laws. In 1870–1 there was a severe but short-lived epidemic of smallpox, and this led, as epidemics always do, to a great increase not only of primary vaccinations but also of revaccinations. From about 1870 to the end of the century, infant vaccination was probably more commonly practised than it has been before or since, and this was the period in which mortality from major smallpox gradually faded from the scene. As the threat of major smallpox has become less menacing, the amount of infant vaccination has become less, and the law has been relaxed from time to time until in 1948 compulsion, which had in fact long been a dead letter, was discontinued. In this matter the amendment of the law really followed the trend of public opinion, for it is extraordinarily difficult to enforce a law for which the justification is not entirely obvious.

It has sometimes been argued that the discontinuance of compulsory infant vaccination was a retrograde step, likely to involve the risk of serious epidemics of major smallpox in this country, but the experience of the past twenty-five years does not really lend support to that view. After all, even the vaccination of all infants is only a partial measure of protection for the community, and any complete scheme would have to include revaccination of all, a procedure which bristles with administrative difficulties. The contrast between the behaviour of minor and major smallpox in the period between the wars does suggest that as a public health measure it is better to use selective vaccination of contacts in instances

* C. Creighton, 1894, Vol. II, p. 584.

of importation of major smallpox rather than to rely on the somewhat broken reed of infant vaccination. This selective vaccination of contacts throws a tremendous burden on the staffs of public health departments but, considering the number of importations of major smallpox which have occurred in recent years, it seems to have been remarkably successful, as is shown in the following table:

	1942	1943	1944	1945	1946	1947	1948
Cases	7	–	16	4	56	78	–
Deaths	–	–	3	–	14	15	–
Importations	1	–	1	1	15	2	–

	1949	1950	1951	1952	1953	1954	1955
Cases	19	8	27	135	30	–	–
Deaths	5	–	10	1	8	–	–
Importations	1	1	1+1*	–	–	–	–

* = Minor

As the Chief Medical Officer of the Ministry of Health says in the *Annual Report* for 1952, 'Previous reports have stressed that the routine vaccination of infants is chiefly to be justified by the protection thereby conferred on the individual. The susceptibility of the community as a whole to epidemic smallpox of either the mild or severe variety cannot be greatly diminished by routine infant vaccination alone.' The Chief Medical Officer goes on to make a plea for more general revaccination, which is, of course, a different matter so far as protection of the community is concerned.

C

5

ASIATIC CHOLERA

CHOLERA is an acute infectious disease due to a micro-organism, the cholera vibrio (discovered by Koch in 1883), which grows in the alimentary canal. The disease is characterized by violent purging, muscular cramps, and rapid collapse. Infection is usually waterborne.

The Indian or Asiatic cholera, which first showed itself on British soil in one or more houses on the Quay at Sunderland in the month of October 1831 was a 'new disease' in a more real sense than anything in this country since the sweating sickness of 1485.*

Cholera is only a name to us in Britain now, and unless some major disaster which dislocates sanitary services overtakes us it seems likely to remain so. Its history is, however, full of interest for several rather unconnected reasons. The menace of cholera was one of the most potent factors in securing the sanitary reforms which have made our towns places so different from what they were at the beginning of the nineteenth century. Cholera had occurred in India before the beginning of the nineteenth century, but for some mysterious reason it began about the year 1817 to spread from its native haunts, not rapidly, but inexorably. The first stage of this first pandemic lasted until 1823, when the disease reached the confines of European Russia. Between 1826 and 1838 it spread to practically the whole of the world between latitude 41° S and 65° N. Thus it showed a power of dispersion almost equal to that of plague or influenza. From the English point of view perhaps the most interesting speculation is why this had never happened before. England had carried on an extensive trade with India for over 200 years, and throughout this period London, at least, must have been just as favourable an environment for an epidemic of cholera

* Creighton, Vol. II, p. 793.

as it was in 1832. Perhaps a partial explanation is that, as cholera has a relatively short incubation period, it could not survive the long sea voyage from India during which an epidemic on shipboard would have burned itself out. The chief explanation seems to be, however, that in 1817 this disease of India acquired a new dynamism which carried it round the world.

Conditions in all the large towns were, at this time, very favourable to the spread of cholera. Much of the drinking water came from wells in the towns themselves which were in close proximity to cesspools. Even when piped water supplies existed, the water was often taken from rivers grossly polluted by human sewage. In London, for example, some of the water companies, between which there was intense competition, derived their supplies direct from the Thames near Westminster. No one realized that the drinking of polluted water was dangerous, and indeed even at the end of the century there were still a few diehards like Creighton who refused to believe that drinking water was an important vehicle of infection. Considering how favourable the conditions were, cholera spread rather slowly.

In Sunderland, with a population of about 18,000, about 400 people were attacked in October–December 1831 and some 200 died. By January 1832 the disease had gained a footing in Newcastle, Gateshead, North Shields, and Houghton le-Spring. The places on Tyneside which were most severely attacked were the low-lying ones near the river, chiefly inhabited by poor industrial workers. It was not until April 1832 that the infection began to show itself obviously in other parts of England. A few suspicious cases occurred at Rotherhithe in the London Dock area in February, and there was a gradual increase until mid-June, when the disease became more severe and affected parishes like St Giles-in-the-Fields in the west end of London. In all there were some 11,000 cases with 5,275 deaths in London in 1832. The most disastrous outbreak in the whole country was at Bilston in the Black Country in August 1832. The population was about 15,000, and in August and September there were some 3,568 cases with 742 deaths. In this first epidemic it is estimated that there were about 22,000 deaths in England and Wales which had, at the time, a population of about 14,000,000.

England was almost free of cholera from 1832 to the second epidemic of 1848–9, but in January 1838 there was an explosive outbreak of cholera-like disease in the Coventry House of Industry with 55 deaths. The severity of the disease suggests that this was true Asiatic cholera.

The second epidemic began in Scotland in October 1848, but did not really reach England until the end of that year. In December there was a terrible outbreak in a large institution for pauper children at Tooting. The school contained about 1,000 children, of whom 300 had the disease and 180 died. In the Spring of 1849 there was little cholera, but in June the epidemic began in real earnest. Once again the Black Country was severely affected, as it had been in 1832, but the outbreaks in Hull and Merthyr Tydfil were even worse. The epidemic chiefly affected manufacturing towns and big ports, and many agricultural counties escaped altogether or had a few unimportant centres of infection. In England and Wales, 53,293 deaths from cholera were registered, and this second epidemic was the most serious of all.

The third visitation was in 1853–4 and, like that of 1831, it began on Tyneside. Again industrial districts were affected chiefly, but some which had been severely affected in one or more of the earlier epidemics escaped. Liverpool, which never escaped, had a moderate epidemic, Merthyr Tydfil had about a quarter of the deaths experienced in 1849, but Plymouth, Hull, Bristol, Manchester, Leeds, and the towns of the Black Country were more or less free of the disease.

This epidemic is notable chiefly because it was the occasion of John Snow's* brilliant inquiry into the source of infection in cholera. Thus thirty years before the discovery of the cholera bacillus he showed clearly that cholera was spread by water contaminated with excrement from cholera sufferers. It is difficult for us now to appreciate the full measure of Snow's achievement, since what he proved seems so obvious, but we must remember that the climate of opinion

* John Snow, 1849.

before the days of bacteriology was completely different from that at the present time. Then, and for many years afterwards, the miasmatic theory of the origin of infectious diseases was the one which was most generally believed. The theory was that soil polluted with excrement or refuse of any kind gave off an atmospheric 'miasma' which was the cause of certain epidemic diseases. There was nothing specific about it, and indeed it was commonly believed that one disease could change into another; for example, even after the clinical distinction between typhoid and typhus had been made, it was commonly believed that one could change into the other. The 'miasmatic' theory was that on which the early movement for sanitary reform was based. In their early years, Chadwick and Simon waged war on all 'filth' indiscriminately and regarded a heap of manure as just as dangerous as a cesspool which was contaminating a well of drinking water. Snow's hypothesis that the excreta of cholera patients contained some specific poison which was transferred to the healthy by drinking water and caused cholera in them was therefore a completely revolutionary one. Perhaps Snow's greatest contribution was, however, his use of the epidemiological method to solve the problem. His inquiry of 1854 into the distribution of cases of cholera around the Broad Street Pump showed that those who had drunk the water from the pump suffered far more than those living in precisely the same conditions and geographical situation who had not drunk the water. He also examined the pump itself and showed how the well had been polluted by the evacuations from sick people near by. At first the General Board of Health did not accept Snow's conclusions, and in a report of 1854 a committee of inquiry into the incident of the Broad Street Pump reported that, 'We do not find it established that the water was contaminated in the manner alleged; nor is there before us any sufficient evidence to show whether inhabitants of the district, drinking from the well, suffered in proportion more than other inhabitants of the district who drank from other sources.' In spite of this official scepticism the theory that water was very important in the spread of cholera received additional confirmation from differences in the incidence of the disease in different households in south London. There were two rival water companies supplying south London. In 1849 both these companies took their supply direct from the grossly polluted Thames in the neighbourhood of Westminster, but before 1854 company A had removed its source of supply to Thames Ditton, higher up the river, whereas company B retained its original source. The pipes of these two companies often interlaced in the same street, so that there was no difference, other than water supply, between most of the houses. It was found that deaths from cholera were 57.1 per 1,000 houses supplied from the polluted source and 11.3 per 1,000 houses supplied from the purer source above Teddington Lock. There had been no such difference in 1849, when the supplies of both companies came from the grossly polluted source.

The last epidemic of cholera in England and Wales was in 1866. It was brought in by emigrants passing from Hull and Grimsby to Liverpool on their way to America. As always, Liverpool had a severe epidemic, with 2,122 deaths, but the only other important centres were Swansea, Neath, Llanelly, Merthyr, Chester, Northwich, a group of towns on the Exe, Portsmouth, and certain parts of east London. The outbreak in London is of particular interest in that three-quarters of the deaths occurred in Whitechapel, Bethnal Green, Poplar, Stepney, Mile End, St Georges-in-the-East, and Greenwich. These districts were supplied by the East London Company from the Old Ford reservoir which was grossly polluted and from which water was supplied without filtration. Sir John Simon said of the outbreak of 1866 in London, 'The area of intense cholera was almost exactly the area of this particular water supply, nearly, if not absolutely, filling it and scarcely, if at all, reaching beyond it'. By 1866, the main drainage scheme of the metropolis had been carried out and all the water companies supplying the western parts had moved their sources of supply much farther up river.

The history of cholera illustrates very well the difficulty of giving complete explanations of epidemiological phenomena. The immediate causation of the English epidemics has been fully explained because the decline of cholera followed so closely the sanitary reforms which safeguarded water supplies from gross pollution with human sewage. The problem which is still unsolved is why the disease relatively suddenly acquired in the nineteenth century an immense power of dispersion which it had apparently never shown before.

6

CONTINUED FEVERS: TYPHUS – ENTERIC (TYPHOID, PARATYPHOID, AND FOOD POISONING)

TYPHUS fever is caused by a member of a group of micro-organisms known as Rickettsia; the organism lives normally in the body louse and the disease is transmitted by the bite of this insect. This mode of transmission was described by Nicolle, Conor, and Conseil in 1911, and five years later da Roche-Lima* isolated the organism (*Rickettsia Prowazeki*). The disease is characterized by severe toxaemia, a high temperature, and a rash.

The enteric fevers are caused by a group of bacteria (*B. typhosus – B. para-typhosus A* and *B*) and as with typhus toxaemia, a high temperature, and a rash are characteristic symptoms. The bacteria gain entry through food or water and live in the large intestine; in consequence enteritis, often with blood in the motion, is an added symptom.

The early histories of typhus and the enteric group of fevers are confused one with another because the clinical distinction between the two diseases was not finally settled in England until Sir William Jenner's treatise which was published in 1893. The distinction between typhus and enteric fever in the Registrar-General's returns of causes of death was first made in 1869, only a short time before typhus disappeared from the English scene.

In earlier times it was appreciated that the 'continued fevers', as they are called, were of different types, but it was thought that one could change into the other. The descriptive names for the two diseases varied from time to time, but perhaps the most commonly used were those adopted by Huxham.† He described a 'slow nervous fever' which

* H. da Roche-Lima, 1916.
† John Huxham, 1755.

was chiefly enteric and a 'putrid malignant fever' which
was chiefly typhus. These were broad distinctions, however,
and many other diseases were, no doubt, included under
both headings.

Although it is not possible to give any comprehensive
picture of the relative importance of typhus and enteric
before the middle of the nineteenth century, it is possible
to make reasonably intelligent guesses and to identify certain famous outbreaks which were almost certainly typhus.

TYPHUS

In the Tudor Period there are at least three accounts of
outbreaks of 'gaol fever' or typhus, originating in the assize
courts – the Black Assizes at Cambridge (1522), at Oxford
(1577), and at Exeter (1586).

At Oxford the Assizes met on 5 and 6 July 1577 and, soon
after, the two Judges, the Sheriff of the County, two Knights,
eight Squires and Justices of the Peace, and many others who
had attended the court fell ill and died. The symptoms were
an acute and rapidly fatal delirium, but no mention is made
of a rash. The disease spread to Merton College and also in
the town, but was soon over.

We catch further glimpses of severe epidemics of typhus
in the Civil War in both the royal and the parliamentary
armies. In 1643 the royal army was holding Reading and
was besieged by Fairfax with an army of 15,000 foot and
3,000 horse. The King and Prince Rupert failed to raise the
siege, but when Fairfax took the town he found it infected,
and his army suffered severely in the ensuing weeks, so much
so that he was unable to pursue his original plan of advanc-
ing on Oxford. The royal army in Oxford was attacked a
little later. Willis,* the great anatomist, was a young man
in Oxford at the time, and he gives a clinical description of
the disease which leaves little doubt that it was typhus. The
victims had an acute fever with delirium or stupor and a
rash. In 1644 there was a severe outbreak at Tiverton which
had recently been occupied by both parliamentary and

* Thomas Willis, 1659.

royalist troops. According to the parish registers 105 of the 8,000 inhabitants were buried in the single month of October 1644, and the total number of burials during the year was 443. These dramatic outbreaks were associated with the miseries of war, as typhus has so often been in human history, but there is little doubt that throughout the seventeenth, eighteenth, and first half of the nineteenth centuries the disease was also a constant visitor to London in particular, and, less frequently, to smaller towns. Throughout the eighteenth century the annual number of deaths in the London Bills from 'Fevers' was usually about 3,000 and sometimes exceeded 7,000. On the whole these deaths slightly exceeded those from smallpox, and fluctuated rather less from year to year. In 1750 there was a Black Assize at the Old Bailey as a result of which there died of fever the Lord Mayor, a Justice of the Common Pleas, a Baron of the Exchequer, and an Alderman, together with many less important persons.

In the latter part of the eighteenth century the great growth of the manufacturing towns of the north produced conditions very favourable to the spread of typhus. The poor lived in grossly overcrowded and insanitary slums, and starvation was never far away. It seems possible that in London typhus may have been a little on the decline. Lettson,* who was one of the first fashionable physicians to visit the poor of London in their homes, wrote in 1773 that, 'In the airy parts of the city and in large open streets, fevers of a putrid tendency rarely arise. . . . In my practice I have attentively observed that at least forty-eight out of fifty of these fevers have existed in narrow courts and alleys'.

Outbreaks of typhus in the nineteenth century were often associated with the great Irish immigrations which followed the potato famines. In England the bad years were 1847–8, and the areas chiefly affected were Lancashire and Cheshire, Liverpool being the town with highest incidence. In the north-western registration district of England there were 9,076 deaths in 1847, and 380 in 1848. In the latter half of the nineteenth century, typhus was declining rapidly. It was

* John C. Lettson, 1774.

still important as a cause of death among the poor of the
great industrial towns, particularly in times of industrial
distress, but by 1870 it had practically disappeared from
southern England and lingered on only in a few of the
northern ports such as Liverpool and Sunderland. In the
twentieth century the disease has occurred only occasionally
in ports as a result of importation from abroad.

Epidemic louse-born typhus is perhaps the best example
of a disease associated with the depths of human misery.

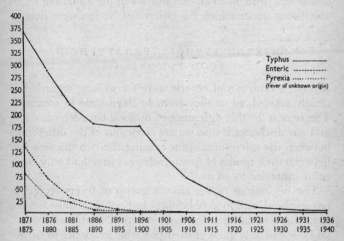

8. *Decline of typhus, enteric, and pyrexia, showing number of deaths per million
of the population in England and Wales, 1871–1940*

Widespread starvation and infestation with body lice are
necessary conditions for the genesis of epidemic typhus, but
when once an epidemic has started it can spread to the
more prosperous members of the community, as it did at
the 'Black Assizes' of the Middle Ages. (Body lice are no
respecters of persons.) Two modern instances may be quoted
to illustrate some essential features of the epidemiology of
typhus. In the First World War the troops on the Western
Front were nearly all infested with body lice, and the louse-
borne disease called trench-fever was common, but the armies

were well-fed and typhus never appeared. In the Second World War typhus broke out in Naples in the winter 1943–4. The epidemic was rapidly brought under control, chiefly by the use of insecticides in powder form. The British troops were also protected by inoculation and only two cases occurred among them, although there were 300 cases amongst the civilian population in the worst week. The epidemic was chiefly remarkable because it was the first in which mass destruction of the insect vector was achieved and the epidemic was brought to an end in spite of the appalling social conditions under which the citizens of Naples were living.

ENTERIC: TYPHOID, PARATYPHOID, FOOD POISONING

Although typhus and enteric were for so long regarded as closely related, to us they seem to have little in common. The reason for this difference of outlook between ourselves and our ancestors is that we are conscious of the differences between the micro-organisms causing the two diseases and between their modes of spread, whereas they had only clinical distinctions to go on.

The beginnings of the enteric group of fevers (typhoid, paratyphoid, and food poisoning) in English history are lost in the mists of the heterogeneous group of 'continued fevers', and one can only guess at their probable incidence in earlier ages. They were probably constantly present in the towns before the Industrial Revolution, but when water and food supplies had a restricted area of distribution, they occurred more as endemic than as epidemic diseases. Epidemics of typhoid would not have had the dramatic quality of the epidemics of typhus associated with the 'Black Assizes', and may well have passed unnoticed against the background of febrile diseases which were the common lot of man.

In the records of admission to the London Fever Hospital during the years 1849 to 1871, cases of enteric were on the increase towards the end of the period. The final disappearance of typhus and the later decline of enteric is shown in Figure 8.

It is difficult to distinguish 'epidemics' of enteric before about the middle of the nineteenth century, but from then on localized epidemics gradually become discernible.

The first outbreak of enteric fever was not numerically large, but will always have historical importance in that it was the inspiration of William Budd's* classical work on the epidemiology of the disease. The epidemic consisted of about eighty cases occurring in the small town of North Tawton, in Devon, and certain neighbouring villages in the summer and autumn of 1839. Budd was a general practitioner in North Tawton at the time, and from his intimate knowledge of the distribution of cases and of the movements of the inhabitants he came to the conclusion that enteric was due to a specific infection which spread from the sick to the healthy, usually in water contaminated by the bowel discharges of the sick. He did not exclude the possibility that the *materies morbi* might pass from the sick to the healthy through the air, but thought that the alimentary route was the more likely. Budd really came to much the same conclusions about enteric as Snow did about cholera, and at very much the same time. Budd, however, did not publish his work until a short time after the appearance of Snow's first paper. Thus both Snow and Budd, by studying the distribution of cases in space and time, established the theory of the mode of transmission of intestinal infections. The final proof of the theory had to wait till the development of bacteriology at the end of the century made it possible to demonstrate the presence of the living organism, which they had only surmised.

The second example is one of the classic instances of an explosive outbreak due to contamination of a public water supply. It occurred at Maidstone in 1897–8, and 1,938 cases in all were reported in a population of about 34,000. To the historian the epidemic is interesting for three reasons. It was the last epidemic in which the explanation of 'miasma' due to soil pollution was seriously considered as a possible alternative to the theory of specific infection of the water supply. It was one of the early epidemics in which

* W. Budd, 1873.

77

bacteriological evidence of faecal pollution of the water supply was produced. A primitive attempt was made to free the water mains from infection by the use of chlorine, which has since become so important a substance for the purification of water supplies.

At this time the water supply of Maidstone was derived from three main sources known as the Farleigh, Cossington, and Boarley supplies. The Farleigh supply was the most subject to human pollution and, just before the epidemic started, hop pickers had been camping near certain springs which contributed to this supply. Most of the cases occurred in the area of the town which received the Farleigh supply and there was a number of cases in the County Asylum which also received this water. The areas supplied from Cossington and Boarley had fewer cases, chiefly in the later stages of the epidemic, and the barracks and prison, supplied from Boarley or a separate well, had no cases at all.

Public water supplies have often been the source of severe outbreaks of typhoid, and the most recent large-scale epidemic due to this cause was that at Croydon between October 1937 and February 1938. In this period there were 310 cases and 43 deaths in a limited area of Croydon. In all probability the outbreak was due to the infection of a deep well at Addington by a workman, a chronic carrier, who was engaged on repair work there in October 1937. While the work was going on untreated water from the well was pumped into the public supply. The cases nearly all occurred among consumers of the 'high level' supply to which the Addington well was one of the two contributory sources. The Croydon outbreak illustrates very well how a single error in the technique of safeguarding the purity of water supplies may be fatal.

Water-borne outbreaks of typhoid have been, perhaps, the largest and most explosive of any, but milk-borne outbreaks are not far behind, and that at Bournemouth and Poole in August and September 1936 is a good modern example. In this epidemic there were 518 cases scattered throughout Bournemouth, Poole, and Christchurch. The water supplies of the three towns were separate, and inquiry showed that all those taken ill in the first wave had drunk raw milk retailed by one firm and distributed by twelve roundsmen. Immediate steps were taken to pasteurize this supply whilst attempts were made to trace the outbreak to its source. Nothing suspicious was found at the headquarters of the retailing firm, but at one of the small holdings (A) among the thirty-seven scattered farms which supplied the retailer it was found that the farmer's wife had been taken ill on 10 August. A diagnosis of typhoid fever was not made until 31 August. At first this appeared to be the source case, but this hypothesis did not quite fit the facts, because twenty-nine cases had occurred in the three towns before the farmer's wife became ill. The small holding occupied by family A was part of what had originally been a farm and two cottages. In all there were five families living there: A already mentioned, B in the cottage next door, and C, D, and E in the original farmhouse. There had been a fatal case of typhoid fever in family B in 1934. These families were all supplied from a well which seemed reasonably satisfactory, but a stream ran past them which aroused suspicion. Careful exploration of the stream above the cottages revealed that about half a mile above them there was a four-inch pipe discharging opaque fluid resembling sewage. It was found that this came from a large house with some sixteen occupants; the effluent from this house discharged into a small impervious tank and the overflow from this discharged via the four-inch pipe into the stream. Bacteriological examinations of the effluent for the presence of typhoid bacillus in September and early October proved negative; but on 16 and 24 October this organism was present in large numbers, but was not found in the stream above the point of entry of the effluent. One occupant of the house who stayed there at intervals and had been staying there in 1934, when the single fatal case occurred in family B, was found to be a chronic intermittent typhoid carrier. The carrier was staying in the house throughout the summer of 1936 up to 10 August, when he went away, and he did not return until 28 September. This story has been told at some length because it is an interesting example of epidemiological detective work. This was the last investigation on which the late Dr Vernon Shaw of the Ministry of Health was engaged, and to tell it again may serve as a small tribute to the work of a distinguished field epidemiologist. As so often happens, there is one link in the chain of evidence which presents a difficulty. How was infection transferred from the stream to the milk? The investigators suggested three possibilities:

1. That water from the stream was used for dairy purposes.
2. That it found its way into the common well which was used for dairy purposes.
3. That A's cows, which were in the habit of drinking at the stream, conveyed the infection. There are three conceivable ways in which this could have happened: (a) by fouling of the udders and teats, (b) by drinking of infected water and subsequent excretion of organisms in the faeces or urine, and (c) by systemic infection of the milk.

Subsequent work suggests that simple mechanical transport of the organisms on the skin of the cows was the most likely mode of infection of the milk.

In the period since the outbreak of the Second World War there have been few important outbreaks of typhoid – one at Aberystwyth in 1946, due to infected ice cream, and one with a high attack rate in an orthopaedic hospital in 1948. Paratyphoid has, however, been widespread from time to time. Outbreaks of paratyphoid are less sharply defined than those of typhoid, and are much more difficult to investigate because of the variability of the incubation period and the mildness and inconstancy of the clinical features of the disease. Figure 9 shows the recent trend of incidence and mortality of the two diseases. For typhoid most of the reduction in mortality has been due to reduction of incidence, but for paratyphoid the deaths hardly rose in 1951 and 1952, even though the disease was more prevalent than it had been since 1941. In both diseases there has, however, been a slight decline in case fatality – possibly due to treatment with a new drug, chloramphenicol. Case fatalities calculated from national figures are always a little doubtful, because it is generally found that in epidemic periods there is an

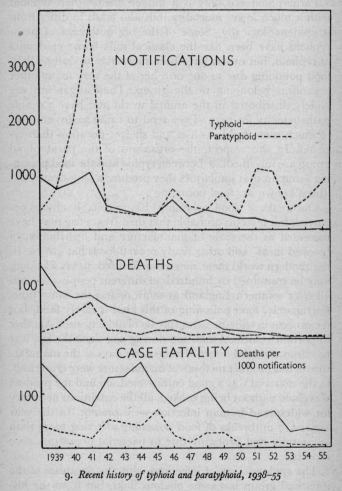

9. *Recent history of typhoid and paratyphoid, 1938–55*

apparent fall in case fatality probably due to better reporting of cases. This can be seen in the figures of paratyphoid in the epidemic year 1941. Recently the numbers of deaths ascribed to these diseases have become so small that rates are misleading for that reason also.

Paratyphoid not only is a milder disease than typhoid with a much lower mortality, but also tends to differ from it epidemiologically. Some of the big outbreaks of paratyphoid have been like the classical milk-borne epidemics of typhoid, but others have been more akin to outbreaks of food poisoning due to one or other of the very many other organisms belonging to the group. These organisms are widely distributed in the animal world and have variable pathogenicity for man. They tend to cause gastro-enteritis of much more sudden onset and shorter duration than typhoid. In this respect, the organisms of the paratyphoid group are intermediate between typhio and the food poisoning group in that sometimes they produce a long-drawn-out illness known as 'food poisoning'.

Outbreaks of 'food poisoning' have probably always occurred, but it seems probable that their frequency may have increased as the scale of manufacture and distribution of 'cooked meat' and other ready-cooked foods has grown. In the modern world meat pies manufactured in, say London, may be consumed by hundreds of different people scattered all over southern England at more or less the same time. Fortunately, food poisoning of this kind is rarely fatal, but it can occur in widespread outbreaks of sudden onset. Another important vehicle of infection during and since the last war has been artificial cream. In the early days of the manufacture of this product methods of manufacture were crude and, as the material was a good culture medium and the product was eaten without being cooked, all the conditions necessary for widespread human infection were present. In the year 1952, 117 outbreaks of food poisoning affecting more than one family and probably due to bacterial organisms were reported.

The epidemiology of infections with any organism of the intestinal group has some obvious links, but from the historical aspect it is perhaps the differences rather than the similarities which are interesting. Cholera had a short history as an important epidemic disease in England and it would appear that in a country of western civilization a profound breakdown of sanitary arrangements would be necessary before cholera could become a serious menace again. Epidemics of typhoid fever are a possible punishment for carelessness in the enforcement of precautions for the protection of water and milk supplies, and outbreaks of infection with food poisoning organisms can occur as a result of some quite minor error of technique in the manufacture of a variety of food products.

7

SUMMER DIARRHOEA OF INFANTS

A CURSORY examination of Figure 10 – a graph of annual
rates of infant mortality (deaths of infants under one year
per 1,000 live births) in England and Wales – shows that,
in the years before the First World War, there were often
great differences in the rates in two successive years. In the
year 1910, for example, the rate fell to the then lowest recorded figure of 105, but in 1911 it rose to 130. A further
scrutiny of the figures of infant mortality shows that these
great fluctuations were associated with variations in the
number of deaths from summer diarrhoea, and that infant
mortality tended to be high in years which had a hot dry
summer and low in years when the summer was cool and
wet (see Figure 10). The last summer in which these rela-
tionships were obvious was that of 1911, but in 1921 there
was a small increase in deaths from diarrhoea associated
with a hot dry summer.

No one knows whether summer diarrhoea, which was a
definite epidemiological entity, was due to a bacterium or
a virus, nor is it known whether the causal organism or
organisms were the same as those which cause fatal diarrhoea in infants nowadays. It is not even absolutely certain
that the disease was an infection at all, though the resem-
blance between it and other infections is so strong that one
feels it must have been.

The zenith of summer diarrhoea was in the later years of
the nineteenth century, and there was at that time a school
of thought which believed that it was, to a great extent, a
product of the Industrial Revolution. Creighton* has, however, pointed out that in London summer diarrhoea of infants can be traced far back in the Bills of Mortality. He

* C. Creighton, 1894.

quotes from a book written by Dr Walter Harris in 1689 on acute diseases of infants:

From the middle of July to the middle of September these epidemic gripes of infants are so common (being the annual heat of the season doth entirely exhaust their strength) that more infants, affected with these, do die in one month than in other three that are gentle.

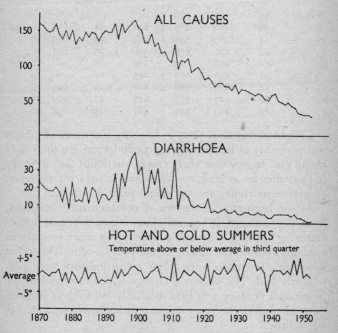

10. *Infant mortality rates from diarrhoea and other causes in England and Wales, 1870–1952*

The story of summer diarrhoea of infants as told in the London Bills is confused by a change in nomenclature which operated between about 1670 and 1720. In the early part of the period deaths from this cause were entered under the heading 'griping of the guts', but throughout the period there was for some reason a gradual transfer to the even less definitive heading of 'convulsions'. A comparison of the weekly returns taken from Creighton for two very hot summers, one at the beginning (1670) and one at the end (1718) of the period, illustrates this point.

Week ending	Con-vulsions	Griping in guts	All causes	Con-vulsions	Griping in guts	All causes	Week ending
		1670			*1718*		
2 Aug.	49	113	470	–	–	–	–
9	38	160	485	226	34	653	12 Aug.
16	44	189	555	239	23	645	19
23	47	222	629	256	25	693	26
30	42	250	629	265	28	668	2 Sept.
6 Sept.	31	253	617	245	27	725	9
13	24	239	586	221	26	653	16
20	38	225	575	213	27	639	23
27	27	150	474	182	24	632	30

Creighton considers that, in London, diarrhoea of infants was probably at its worst in the period 1720–40, the era of cheap gin. In any case there can be no doubt that in every hot summer for at least 300 years before 1911 there was an enormous mortality among infants from diarrhoea.

At the beginning of the era of comprehensive statistics, from 1837 onward, it became obvious that the great manufacturing towns of the north suffered even more severely in epidemics of summer diarrhoea than did London. The towns where many women were employed in industry were particularly bad. The only real change which occurred in the nineteenth century was that mortality fell slightly in London, whereas in the great manufacturing towns it tended to rise a little.

In the year 1911 no less than 31,900 deaths among infants under a year were ascribed to diarrhoea and enteritis, and in 1956 only 319 were reported. Besides this enormous decline in the absolute number of deaths, there has been a change in the seasonal distribution. In 1911 nearly all deaths from diarrhoea and enteritis in infants occurred in the late summer and early autumn, whereas nowadays the deaths from this cause are much more evenly distributed throughout the year.

Nowadays fatal diarrhoea tends to occur in outbreaks in institutions where a number of young babies are congregated. A great deal of work has been done on the bacteriology of these outbreaks, and the general conclusion seems to be that they are generally but not always due to particular kinds of bacillus coli. The subject is a difficult one, because other kinds of bacillus coli are normal and harmless inhabitants of the human intestine. It seems almost as though a disease which now occurs only as an occasional, if dangerous, visitor in institutions was formerly a nation-wide scourge in every hot summer. It is interesting to speculate on possible explanations for this; one which has been suggested is that the decline in summer diarrhoea may have been associated with the decline in the use of horses. This theory involves the assumption that the disease was largely fly-borne and that the disappearance of the heaps of manure, a splendid breeding ground for flies, from our cities so reduced the fly population that the great summer epidemics ceased. Perhaps all one can say is that the theory seems plausible but cannot now be proved or disproved.

Death rates are impersonal things, and it may be helpful to summarize the history of fatal diarrhoea in infants under one year in England and Wales by giving total numbers of deaths in some representative hot summers:

Year	Deaths from diarrhoea	Deaths from all causes	Ratio between deaths from diarrhoea and deaths from all causes
1911	31,900	114,600	1:3.6
1921	11,705	70,250	1:6
1933	3,558	36,960	1:10
1949	1,963	23,882	1:12

Thus the number of deaths in 1911 from diarrhoea alone was 8,000 more than the deaths from all causes in 1949. Moreover, the proportion of infantile deaths caused by diarrhoea has decreased from 1 in 3.6 in 1911 to 1 in 12 in 1949.

8

THROAT DISTEMPERS: SCARLET FEVER – DIPHTHERIA

LIKE the chapters on typhus and typhoid fevers, this chapter concerns two diseases which we now know to have different causes. Scarlet fever and diphtheria have in common the symptom of a sore throat, and the early history of the two diseases is therefore confused.

Before the days of bacteriology, a clinical distinction between these two types of sore throat rested largely on the later symptoms, which might or might not arise. In trying to distinguish the two diseases in the early accounts of epidemics we have, therefore, to rely entirely on the prominent symptoms and signs. For scarlet fever these are the sore throat and the rash, but we have to remember that many patients with a streptococcal sore throat do not develop a rash. They have not got 'scarlet fever', because the rash and the 'scarlet' are synonymous, but they have a disease which is in other respects identical, and they may indeed have acquired their infection from a patient who has typical 'scarlet' fever. Kidney disease with dropsy used to be a common complication of scarlet fever. The distinguishing marks of diphtheria are the sore throat, sometimes associated with paralysis, particularly paralysis of the soft palate which leads to regurgitation of fluids through the nose, and obstruction of the larynx, popularly known as 'croup'. Unfortunately Home, writing in 1765, thought that 'croup' was a separate disease, and this view persisted so long that 'diphtheria' and 'croup' still appeared as separate headings in the Registrar-General's returns even as late as 1910. The diphtheria bacillus was first isolated by Löffler* in 1884, though it had previously been found by Klebs in 1883.

The final proof that scarlet fever was due to infection with

* F. Löffler, 1884.

haemolytic streptococci came relatively late in the history of bacteriology — in 1924 — when the Dicks* produced the disease experimentally in a woman volunteer. Streptococci are spheroid or ovoid organisms arranged in short or long chains. When grown on a medium that contains blood, some specimens have the power to lyse the blood, thus leaving a clear colourless circle around the colony of bacteria; such streptococci are known as haemolytic streptococci.

SCARLET FEVER (SCARLATINA)

SEVENTEENTH AND EIGHTEENTH CENTURIES

From the early accounts of severe throat distempers it is extremely difficult to decide whether the observer was describing a severe form of streptococcal sore throat or diphtheria. Sydenham† described febris scarlatina in 1675, and he regarded it as a mild disease which was rarely fatal, but Fothergill‡ (1748) and Huxham§ both described outbreaks of very severe sore throats with many deaths. Fothergill was writing of London and Huxham of Plymouth. The title of Fothergill's little book is *An Account of the Sore Throat Attended with Ulcers*, and on the title page of the second edition this is described as 'a disease (which) hath of late years appeared in this city and . . . in several parts of the nation'. In his preface Fothergill refers to a simple inflammation of the tonsils which is common and trivial, but goes on to say that 'a disease hath of late years appeared in this city (London), in many of the neighbouring villages, and according to the best information I have been able to secure, in several parts of the nation, which, tho' it may be taken for a common sore throat, or inflammation of the tonsils, by those who are unacquainted with it, is of a very different nature.' Osler‖ quotes Fothergill in his historical note on diphtheria, but Fothergill's notes of cases suggest that he was describing a severe form of scarlet fever rather than diphtheria. It is, however, impossible to say whether or not he

* G.F. and G.H. Dicks, 1934.   † T. Sydenham, 1676.
‡ J. Fothergill, 1748.   § John Huxham, 1755.
‖ W. Osler, 1920.

may have been describing diphtheria as well. Huxham's description also seems to refer to severe scarlet fever rather than to diphtheria. Both Fothergill and Huxham make frequent reference to a skin rash, and Huxham speaks of generalized dropsy.

At the end of the eighteenth century Willan* gave a remarkably good and complete description of scarlet fever in his book on cutaneous diseases. He described three types:

1. Scarlatina simplex with a rash and no sore throat.
2. Scarlatina anginosa with a rash and a sore throat which might be very severe.
3. Scarlatina maligna which was a very severe form of scarlatina anginosa with sloughing of the soft tissues of the throat and mouth and profound toxaemia.

He pointed out that cases of very different degrees of severity could occur in the same household and that the sore throat occurred without the rash. He states that the severe form of the disease was the leading epidemic disease in London in 1786. From 1804 to 1816 Bateman† kept records of the diseases of London based on his experience as physician to the Public Dispensary and consulting physician to the Fever Institution in London. In Autumn 1807 and again in 1808 he wrote that scarlatina was generally mild, presenting the eruption with a slight sore throat. In the autumn of 1814 he wrote as follows:

The scarlatina has been, in all cases, accompanied by sore throat, in the adults, indeed, in two or three families, the throat, as is usual, was the only seat of the disease, as the rash did not appear on the skin. Under the cool treatment, which, however is often imperfectly accomplished in the close and crowded apartments of the poor, these cases have uniformly done well.

Bateman also mentions dropsy following scarlet fever.

In the light of our modern knowledge of streptococcal sore throat is seems clear that bad epidemics occurred in the eighteenth century, that there were quite long intervals between them, and that sometimes in the early years of the

* R. Willan, 1798–1808.   † Thomas Bateman, 1819.

nineteenth century – probably about 1803 – the disease became milder, though it was still common.

NINETEENTH AND TWENTIETH CENTURIES

The mild phase of scarlet fever lasted until about 1830, but from then on the disease began to increase in severity again, and in the first two and a half years (1836–9) of registration the number of deaths attributed to this cause was considerable. In 1840 the number of deaths nearly doubled and, for

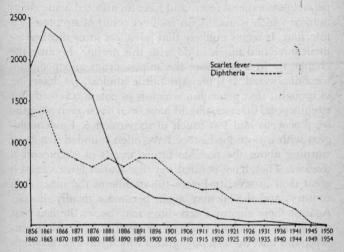

11. *Deaths from scarlet fever and diphtheria per million living under fifteen years of age, 1856–1954*

a generation after, scarlet fever was the leading cause of death amongst the infectious diseases of childhood. Creighton says of this period: 'The enormous number of deaths from scarlatina during some thirty or forty years in the middle of the nineteenth century will appear in history as one of the most remarkable things in our epidemiology'. The year of highest mortality was 1863 when the death rate of children under fifteen was 3,966 per million living. In 1863 there were just over 30,000 deaths from scarlet fever, and in 1953 there were 27.

Figure 11 shows the trend of death rates from scarlet fever of children under fifteen from the time when scarlet fever and diphtheria were separated in the statistical returns to the present. The marked decline of mortality began in the quinquennium 1866–70 and has continued pretty steadily ever since. No satisfactory explanation of this decline has ever been offered, but it may be due to a diminution of virulence of the haemolytic streptococcus, as a similar fall has occurred in other streptococcal diseases such as erysipelas and puerperal fever, and has also affected acute rheumatism which is usually an indirect result of streptococcal infection. It seems unlikely that advances in medical treatment have had much to do with this decline, because the change set in long before the sulpha drugs and penicillin were discovered. It is perhaps a little ironical, yet deserving of thought, that penicillin, which is so potent a remedy for streptococcal diseases, should have been discovered after the streptococcus had lost much of its virulence. Epidemiologists with a taste for history have often sounded a note of warning about the possible future trends of streptococcal diseases. They have pointed out that scarlet fever varied a great deal in severity before the middle of the nineteenth century, and that it may again become a deadly disease. Against these gloomy forebodings may be set the fact that the decline in severity has gone on steadily for nearly a century, and that we now have drugs which will kill the streptococci without hurting the patient.

DIPHTHERIA

EARLY HISTORY

Some examples of outbreaks of severe sore throat occurring in the eighteenth century have been given already. Most of the accounts quoted have suggested that the disease described was scarlet fever rather than diphtheria, but there are others in which the description is more like diphtheria than scarlet fever.

In 1750 John Starr of Liskeard in Cornwall described an outbreak of severe sore throat in which the prominent symp-

toms and signs were agonized breathing and an inflammation of the throat with the formation of membrane. In one
case, that of a child, the father pulled from the child's mouth
a complete membraneous cast of the wind-pipe.

Although Huxham's* descriptions of the disease in Plymouth about 1751 seem to refer to severe scarlet fever, he
also mentions membrane in the wind-pipe, which suggests
diphtheria rather than scarlet fever. All one can say about
this difficult early period is that the evidence seems to suggest that severe scarlet fever was a more prevalent disease
than diphtheria, but that diphtheria did occur.

It seems certain that diphtheria was not an important
disease in England in the first half of the nineteenth century,
though there were probably small outbreaks, e.g. Ashford
(Kent) 1817, Lifton (Devon) 1852.

In France, however, it was important, and the modern
description of the disease was given by Bretonneau of Tours
in 1821 in a paper to the Academy.

MODERN HISTORY

The modern history of diphtheria in England begins with
the wave of prevalence which started about 1855. Simon's†
second report to the Privy Council for the year 1859 has a
section of 160 pages about it. He says that the disease was
almost unknown to British doctors until 1855, but in the
four years since then it had become widespread. As is usual
when an epidemic disease which has been rare becomes
common, importation from abroad was blamed, and at first
diphtheria was known as 'the Boulogne sore-throat'. If it
was indeed imported it seems to have spread far and fast.
In 1855–6 epidemics were reported from places so widely
scattered as Launceston (Cornwall), Spalding (Lincolnshire), Thame (Oxfordshire), Billericay (Essex), Ash (Kent),
and many other places. In 1859 the 9,587 deaths ascribed
to the disease were scattered throughout England and
Wales.

At first diphtheria was overshadowed by scarlet fever as
a cause of death among children, but in the quinquennium

* J. Huxham, 1755.   † Sir John Simon, 1860.

1886–90 it took the lead (see Figure 11) and remained a leading cause of death in children up to 1941.

When epidemic diphtheria first appeared it tended to affect rural areas more than urban, but in the second half of the nineteenth century and the first forty years of the twentieth there was a gradual change, so that in the decennium 1871–80 the rural areas had a death rate only slightly higher than that of the urban, and by 1939 the County Boroughs had a substantially higher rate than the Rural Districts. In the early years of the twentieth century diphtheria tended to kill children under school age more than

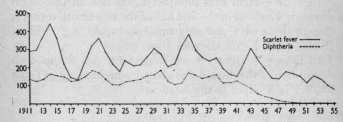

12. *Notifications of scarlet fever and diphtheria in England and Wales per 100,000 of the population, 1911–55*

older children, but here again there was a gradual change, and in 1938 diphtheria was the chief cause of death among children aged 5–9.

The trend of mortality among children is shown in Figure 11. After the first outburst in the sixties the death rate remained more or less stable at about 800 per million living until about 1900; then there was a slow fall to about 300 in 1921–5, and thereafter a period of stability until 1940. Antitoxin was first used in treatment in England in 1895, and it seems reasonable to suppose that the reduction in mortality between 1896–1900 and 1921–5 was chiefly due to the improvement in the treatment of the established disease. More efficient treatment saved many lives, but it had no effect on incidence, and the graph of annual notifications (Figure 12) showed fluctuations but no consistent downward trend. The diphtheria bacillus itself lives chiefly

in the throat and nose of the host, causing a local inflammation, but it also produces a powerful poison (toxin) which
circulates in the host's blood and causes the more serious
symptoms and signs of diphtheria. The antitoxin which is
so effective in the treatment of established disease is an
agent for 'passive' immunization and can be used to secure
temporary protection against catching the disease. It is
made by the 'active' immunization of horses, and the serum
from the immunized horse, which is rich in antibodies, is
injected into the person to be protected. Passive immunization is only temporary, and clearly some safe method of
producing the 'active' immunization of man was always
likely to be far more effective in controlling the disease than
'passive' immunization. Bacteriologists recognized this quite
early, and in 1913 the first effective diphtheria prophylactic
was produced. Unfortunately this was not absolutely safe,
and it was not until 1923 that an effective and safe antigen
for the protection of man was produced. In the late twenties
and the thirties a certain amount of active immunization
of children was done in Britain but was insufficient to influence diphtheria as a disease of the community. In other
countries, however, notably in the United States and Canada,
a great deal was done, and it became clear that active
immunization of large numbers of children could reduce the
incidence of and mortality from diphtheria in the community. In 1940 the Ministry of Health, inspired by Sir William
Jameson, its chief medical officer, embarked on a campaign
to popularize the immunization of all children against diphtheria. The mortality from diphtheria from 1911 to 1955 is
shown in Figure 13, in which it is compared with those of
measles and whooping-cough.

In 1941, an extremely rapid decline of both incidence and
mortality of diphtheria began, and has continued until the
present time. In a dozen years diphtheria has become a very
rare disease, so much so that a generation of doctors is
growing up who have never seen a patient suffering from it.
The recent history of diphtheria in the countries of Western
Europe has been quite different. Virulent diphtheria came
with the German armies, and in the occupied countries

there was a steep rise in the death rate from diphtheria during the years of the Second World War. In Holland, for example, the death rate rose from 0.9 per 100,000 living in 1939 to 46 per 100,000 in 1945. Since then it has declined. In 1945 there were 4,270 deaths and in 1952 only 173.

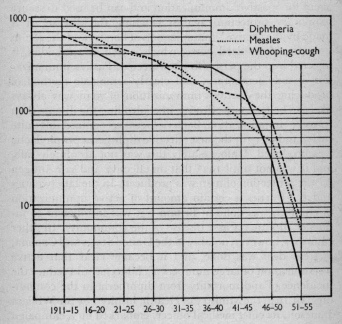

13. *Decline of mortality in England and Wales from diphtheria, measles, and whooping-cough, 1911–55*

Memories are short, and there is no doubt that it is now very much more difficult to persuade parents to have their children immunized than it was in 1941. This is a disturbing state of affairs, but the wholesale immunization of children has had one unexpected result which makes it a little less disturbing than it might at first sight appear to be. In theory there is no reason why immunization against the toxin of the diphtheria bacillus should have any effect on the population of diphtheria bacilli. One might reasonably expect that the number of healthy human carriers would increase as the number of cases of overt disease diminished. There is some evidence, however, that in fact the population of diphtheria bacilli has declined *pari passu* with the decline of the disease. Small epidemics of diphtheria do, however, still occur, and are particularly dangerous because the disease is now so uncommon that it is often some time before a correct diagnosis is made.

Diphtheria is the most convincing example of a disease which can be controlled by artificial active immunization, and any reasonable person must be convinced that, in England, the hard work of public health officers has been the most important factor in determining its virtual disappearance in the last twelve years. Their achievement has been considerable. In 1941 there were 50,000 notified cases with 1,622 deaths, and in 1956 there were 37 cases with 6 deaths.

9

MEASLES AND WHOOPING-COUGH

MEASLES and whooping-cough are not particularly alike in their symptoms, but they have other affinities which justify their sharing of a chapter. Perhaps the most obvious of these is that nearly all of us have at some time in our lives had both diseases, and it seems likely that most of our ancestors had much the same experience. From the notification returns it would appear that measles is about three times as common as whooping-cough, but whooping-cough is more difficult to diagnose because the characteristic 'whoop' is not a constant symptom, and so the returns are less complete than are those of measles. Both diseases still have their dangers for young children, though they have become much less dangerous in the twentieth century. In both, the complications, rather than the original diseases, cause death and disability.

Measles is caused by a virus, but little is known of its size or shape. It has been cultivated in tissue from a chick embryo, and several species of monkey can be infected with it. In contrast with some other viruses, for example, that of influenza, the virus of measles appears to have remained stable for hundreds of years. When a susceptible person is exposed to infection he almost invariably develops measles and the resulting immunity is nearly always complete and long lasting. Because so many people have had an attack of measles, serum prepared from an ordinary blood bank is rich in antibodies, and this property has been used to modify the attack in weakly children after a known exposure to infection. Nowadays the usual procedure is to give an injection of γ globulin (that fraction of the serum protein which contains the antibodies) to the exposed child about five days after exposure. The object is to produce a modified attack which will save the weakly child from a severe illness but will at the same time produce lasting immunity.

Whooping-cough is caused by a small bacillus discovered by Bordet and Gengou* in 1906. An attack of the disease usually produces lasting immunity, but second attacks are not quite so rare as are those of measles. Many attempts have been made to produce a safe and effective vaccine to protect against whooping-cough, and modern vaccines will produce immunity in a good proportion of children.

On the whole the bacteriology of these two diseases is not important to an understanding of their history. The diagnosis depends and always has depended chiefly on signs and symptoms, and these are sufficiently characteristic to enable us to trace their history reasonably well. Measles is a febrile illness which starts like a severe cold and has a blotchy rash which comes out on the third or fourth day. In whooping-cough the characteristic is the cough, which becomes more and more paroxysmal, each paroxysm ending with the characteristic crowing inspiration or 'whoop'.

MEASLES

EARLY HISTORY

The name mézils seems to have been used first by John of Gaddesden (1280–1361), who applied it both to measles and to certain leprous lesions. In the Arabic writings variolae (smallpox) and morbilli (measles) are an inseparable pair, and the same is true of 'smallpox and mezils' in the writings of Tudor times. At that time measles was generally thought to be a mild form of smallpox, though the severe form of haemorrhagic smallpox was also confused with it. Probably by 1620, when the Parish Clerks first returned measles under a separate heading in the Bills, the distinction between smallpox and measles was reasonably well understood. In the first series of London Bills from 1629 to 1660 the deaths vary from only 2 in 1630 to 153 in 1656. In the next series the numbers of deaths became greater, 311 in 1664 and 295 in 1670. The epidemic of 1670 is notable because it gave Sydenham† his opportunity, and his clinical description would seem quite at home in a modern textbook. There was

* J. Bordet and O. Gengou, 1906.   † T. Sydenham, 1676.

another bad epidemic in 1674 with 795 deaths in the Bills, and then a long interval of low mortality until 1705–6 when nearly 800 deaths were returned for the two years. In this early period the bad epidemics apparently came at long intervals. In the eighteenth century epidemics in London became more frequent, and by the middle of it were occurring every other year or every three years but not with the biennial regularity which was so prominent a feature of measles in London in the nineteenth century and the early years of the twentieth.

In the early years of the nineteenth century smallpox began to decline as a common cause of death in children, and measles and whooping-cough became more prominent, though it is difficult to say whether the number of deaths increased absolutely or only relatively. In this period, immediately before the introduction of universal registration of births and deaths, the Bills are notoriously incomplete. In the first four complete years of registration 1838–42 the common infectious diseases of childhood had the following mean annual death rates per million living at all ages:

Scarlet fever	797
Measles	539
Whooping-cough	504

Diphtheria had not yet been separated from scarlet fever, but as we have already seen it seems unlikely that it was an important cause of death at this time. Scarlet fever was just beginning to assume the prominence which became obvious in the sixties and seventies, and measles and whooping-cough had rates about the same as they had in the second half of the century.

MODERN HISTORY

The trend of the death rate of children under fifteen from 1851 to 1955 is shown in Figure 14. At the beginning of the period measles had a slightly higher rate than that of whooping-cough, but the rate for measles began to decline later, and even in the early years of the First World War it was very nearly the same as it had been in 1871–5. Since

1915, in which year there was a bad epidemic, there has been a rapid fall in mortality. In 1915 16,445 deaths resulted from measles, and in 1955 only 176, in spite of the fact that there were nearly half a million notifications (the disease was not notifiable in 1915).

There is no evidence that the incidence of measles has decreased at all. It has been generally notifiable only since 1940, and the annual notification rates since then are shown

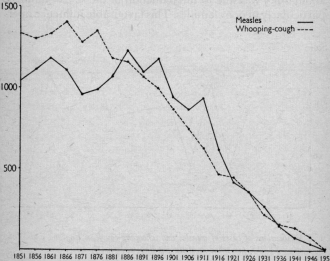

14. *Deaths of children in England and Wales under fifteen from measles and whooping-cough per million of the population, 1851–1955*

in Figure 15. Incidence varies enormously in different years; for example, there were about 160,000 notifications in 1946 and about 600,000 in 1951. The reduction in mortality has, therefore, been entirely due to the fact that the disease has become less fatal than it used to be.

The reasons for the decline of the fatality of measles are probably complex. It began to fall many years before there were any really effective drugs for the treatment of the fatal complications. Deaths from measles have always tended to occur in young children, particularly in those between six months and two years old. Those under six months have antibodies derived from their mother and so are less liable to develop the disease than slightly older children, and children over two have a stronger hold on life than the very young. Anything, therefore, which will tend to postpone the age of attack will tend to make the disease less mortal. It seems likely that much of the reduction from about 1915 to about 1935 was due to the reduction in the size of families, particularly of poor families. This favourable influence oper-

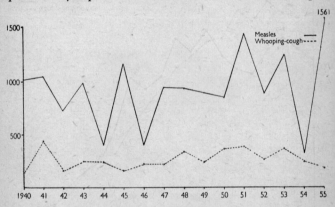

15. *Notifications of cases of measles and whooping-cough in England and Wales per 100,000 of the population, 1940–55*

ated in two ways. The older children who go to school pick up infectious diseases there, and bring them back to their younger brothers and sisters. When there are many younger brothers and sisters in the population measles will tend to occur at an early age and will tend to be more dangerous. In addition to the danger of infection at an early age in the large family there is the obvious factor of poor feeding and all the other factors which make up the complex of poor social conditions. The total effect of these influences on mortality from measles was examined in the Registrar-General's Decennial Supplement 1931, p. 167. The mortality from measles of children aged one in social class V was nearly twenty times that of children of the same age in social class I.

There is no convincing evidence in the national figures indicating that the sulpha drugs and penicillin have had much influence on mortality. The decline has been a little steeper since about 1935 than it was before, but not very markedly so. Passive immunization with serum or γ globulin has never been used on a sufficient scale to have any influence on national figures.

In contrast to diphtheria, measles is a disease in which changes in social conditions rather than advances in methods of prevention or treatment have been the important factor in determining the decline of mortality. The decline of virulence of the haemolytic streptococcus which was discussed in the chapter on scarlet fever, has also had something to do with it, because infections with haemolytic streptococci used to be common and fatal complications of the disease.

WHOOPING-COUGH

Creighton* says that there is singularly little reference to whooping-cough in early medical writings, and suggests that a possible reason may be that it was generally left to the management of parents and nurses and also that it may have been thought of as a complication of other diseases rather than as a disease in its own right. There is, however, a reference to 'the kink' in a medieval prescription book. The first medical description of an epidemic was that given by Baillou† of Paris in 1578. Sydenham‡ mentions it under the name pertussis 'which we call hooping-cough' but always in association with another disease – in one instance with measles and in another with influenza. There is one description, written by a mother to her husband in 1661, which will arouse a little wave of sympathy in the heart of any modern parent who has nursed a child through the disease: 'I am in a sad condition for my poor children, who are all so trobled with the chincofe that I am afraid it will kill them. There is many dye out in this town, and many abroad that we heare of. I am fane to have a candell stand by me to goo

* C. Creighton, 1894.   † Baillou of Paris, 1578.
‡ T. Sydenham, 1676.

in too them when the fitt comes.' In a later letter: 'Moll is much the worst. They have such fits that it stopes theare wind, and puts me to such fits and feares that I am not myselfe.' In a third letter the children are said to be better and the mother asks her husband to bring 'a paper of lozenges for them'. It seems clear that in the seventeenth century whooping-cough was a common and distressing malady of children, just as it is now, but as a cause of death it was overshadowed by other diseases, particularly by small-pox, and so did not attract much notice from doctors.

In the Bills of Mortality 'hooping-cough and chincough' do not achieve a separate heading until 1701 and for fifteen years the deaths returned are only units; in 1715 they rise to tens and by the end of the century are counted in hun-dreds – in 1780 for example 573 deaths were ascribed to 'hooping-cough'. It seems probable that in the early part of the century many deaths really due to whooping-cough were returned under the indefinite heading of 'convulsions'.

In the early years of the nineteenth century measles and whooping-cough together began to replace smallpox as the principal killing disease of young children. In Glasgow, Robert Watt* demonstrated this by a painstaking examina-tion of the Parish Registers, and published his findings as an appendix to his *Treatise on the History, Nature, and Treat-ment of Chincough*. Although in most years smallpox killed fewer children than measles and whooping-cough, it still surpassed them from time to time when it became epidemic. In the first six months of registration in England and Wales the deaths from the principal causes of death among chil-dren were as follows:

Convulsions	10,729
Smallpox	5,811
Measles	4,732
Whooping-cough	3,004
Scarlatina	2,550

An epidemic of smallpox was just beginning at this time but had not reached its full force in London. In London, in contrast with the rest of England and Wales, the number

* Robert Watt, 1813.

of deaths from measles and from whooping-cough separately greatly exceeded the number of deaths from smallpox.

The trend of mortality from whooping-cough in children under fifteen from 1851 to 1955 is shown in Figure 14. From 1851 to 1880 it altered little, and was rather higher than that of measles, but it began to decline rather earlier than did the death rate of measles, and in the quinquennium 1886–90 it fell below that of measles and remained below until the quinquennium 1921–5. Since then now one disease and now the other has been the more important, their relative importance depending chiefly on incidence.

Of late years the death rate of whooping-cough has been consistently higher than that of measles, but in 1955 it was the same, that is, 24 per million living under 15. The actual number of deaths attributed to measles in 1955 was 176 and to whooping-cough 88, but a higher proportion of the deaths from whooping-cough occurred in infants under a year old.

The same influences which have led to the decline of mortality from measles have resulted in the decline of mortality from whooping-cough. As we have seen, mortality from whooping-cough began to fall rather earlier than that of measles, and it may be that this is due to the fact that whooping-cough tends to have its highest mortality at a rather younger age than measles. In 1931 mortality from whooping-cough of babies one year old was very much higher in children of social class V (i.e. the R.G.'s lowest social grade). The difference was nearly but not quite as great as in the case of measles. It would be interesting to be able to trace the history of the case fatality (deaths and notifications) of these two diseases further back than 1940, but unfortunately they were not generally notifiable before then. In 1940, one in every seventy cases of whooping-cough died. In 1955 only one death occurred for every nine hundred cases. The recent history of death rates for whooping-cough and measles (Figure 14) shows that the trend in recent years has been similar for both diseases. The fall has been particularly steep since 1947, and this may have been due to the more effective treatment of complications by penicillin and other antibiotics. There is no sign in the statistics of notifications of any consistent downward trend of incidence, but now that an effective vaccine has been made for whooping-cough there seems no reason why a reduction in incidence of the disease should not be achieved. It is not likely that the dramatic results which followed diphtheria immunization will be obtainable, because it is usually easier to prepare a really effective prophylactic for a 'toxin' disease like diphtheria than for a bacterial disease like whooping-cough. Such a vaccine must be given early in life, because whooping-cough is such a severe and distressing disease in the very young. Nothing has been said of the disability which follows these two diseases because it is impossible to make any numerical estimate. There is no doubt, however, that in spite of their decline in severity, both diseases still cause a great deal of chronic illness in children, and that anything which can be done to postpone the age of attack will reduce the likelihood of permanent disability.

In summarizing the history of these two common infectious diseases of children, it is justifiable to treat them together because the general lines of their history have been much the same. Both have been extremely common for at least two hundred years and probably for much longer. Hardly anyone goes through life without having measles, and there is little prospect of any change in that almost universal incidence. Whooping-cough is and always has been rather less common, and it is possible that a really effective vaccine may be available in the near future. Throughout the nineteenth and early twentieth centuries both were serious killing diseases of children, particularly of very young children, but their importance in this respect has declined. At first the decline seems to have been due chiefly to non-specific factors; to improvements in social conditions and especially to the reduction in the size of families. Very recently improvements in the medical treatment of complications have hastened the decline of mortality. So far specific methods for prevention have had little effect on the incidence or mortality of either disease, but there is a prospect that a vaccine may effect the future history of whooping-cough.

10

EPIDEMIC DISEASES OF THE CENTRAL NERVOUS SYSTEM: CEREBROSPINAL FEVER – ANTERIOR POLIOMYELITIS – ENCEPHALITIS LETHARGICA

EPIDEMIC diseases which have signs and symptoms chiefly affecting the central nervous system are conveniently grouped together because their precise differentiation has come relatively late in history and has depended on the development of clinical neurology in the nineteenth century and that of bacteriology in the late nineteenth and twentieth centuries.

These diseases have probably never been common in the sense that plague, typhus, and smallpox were once common or that some of the infectious diseases of childhood are now. It is always possible, therefore, that epidemics may have occurred in earlier days and have been overshadowed by the more common diseases. In the Restoration period, for example, there are accounts of 'fevers' by Willis* and by Sydenham† which epidemiologists of our own time have tried to identify with cerebrospinal fever or with encephalitis lethargica. In 1661, Willis described a 'fever' in which sometimes frenzy and sometimes coma were prominent symptoms; the disease usually affected children and fits occurred. Sydenham also gave an account of this fever in 1661, and Goodall‡ in his little book on the history of infectious diseases suggests that it may have been cerebrospinal fever. A few years later, in 1673–4, Sydenham reported 'comatose' fevers. The original accounts are, however, extremely confusing because they mention so many symptoms not specially connected with the central nervous system, and it would be possible to make some sort of case

* T. Willis, 1659.   † T. Sydenham, 1676.
‡ C. Goodall, 1661.

for regarding these fevers as any one of a number of other diseases, with typhus perhaps the most probable.

On the whole, therefore, it is an interesting but unprofitable exercise to spend much time on the early history of the epidemic diseases of the central nervous system, and in the study of individual diseases the starting-point will be the first modern description.

From time to time there has been confusion between the three diseases, and indeed between them and other diseases.

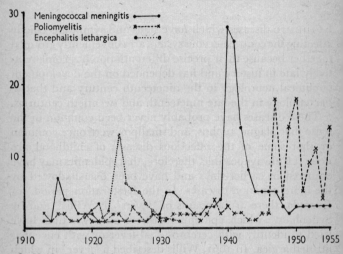

16. *Notifications of epidemic diseases of the central nervous system in England and Wales per 100,000 of the population, 1913–55*

For example, when widespread epidemics of poliomyelitis began in 1910 and 1911 they were at first mistaken for epidemics of cerebrospinal fever, and when encephalitis lethargica appeared in 1918 it was mistaken for a severe form of food poisoning, known as botulism, which also affects the central nervous system. Clear-cut cases of these diseases are not difficult to distinguish one from another, but there are many atypical cases in which it is difficult to make an exact diagnosis. For these reasons statistics are inevitably inexact. They do, however, give a general picture of incidence and mortality which is reasonably accurate (Figure 16).

In all three diseases the number of persons who become infected with the causal organism far exceeds the number who develop obvious disease. The bacteriologists have shown that this is true of cerebrospinal fever and poliomyelitis but, as the organism which causes encephalitis lethargica has never been directly demonstrated, the theory that healthy carriers are important rests only on analogy with the other diseases. Healthy carriers and patients with mild and atypical disease are, of course, important reservoirs of infection in many epidemic diseases, but they are particularly important in the epidemic diseases of the central nervous system.

CEREBROSPINAL FEVER

Cerebrospinal fever (spotted fever, meningococcal meningitis) is an acute inflammation of the membraneous coverings of the brain caused by a bean-shaped organism which is usually found in pairs within the cells in the cerebrospinal fluid. The meningococcus was discovered by Weichselbaum* in 1887, but the disease had been distinguished clinically long before, though it may have been confused with meningitis due to other organisms. The main symptoms and signs are intense headache, vomiting, high temperature, and stiffness of the neck so severe that the head becomes bent backwards by the spasm of the muscles and is held in that position. These are signs and symptoms of any form of acute meningitis, and the final diagnosis depends on examination of the cerebrospinal fluid. It so happens, however, that epidemics of very acute meningitis are always due to the meningococcus, and we can assume that those described before bacteriological confirmation was possible were cerebrospinal fever. The meningococcus is found in the secretions from the nose of perfectly healthy people, particularly in times of epidemics, and it seems that the disease cerebrospinal fever is a rare manifestation of infection with the meningococcus.

* A. Weichselbaum, 1887.

The first identifiable description of an epidemic was given by Viesseux* and related to an epidemic at Geneva in 1805, though, as has been said, it is not certain whether or no some of the 'nervous' fevers described by the physicians of the Restoration period may have been cerebrospinal fever. In the early stages of its history it was noticed that the disease tended to be associated with troops living in over-crowded barracks. There were several examples of this among the French garrisons in the Napoleonic wars. Hirsch† writing in 1886 divided the history of the disease in the world as a whole into four periods: (1) 1805–30, (2) 1837–50, (3) 1854–75, (4) 1876–86, but apart from two rather doubt-ful small epidemics in England, one on Dartmoor in 1807, and one at Sunderland in 1830, it did not affect that country until 1865 and even then not very much. In writing about this period, Simon, medical officer of the Privy Council, describes cerebrospinal fever as 'a disease which we in England had hitherto hardly heard named and which on the continent had but recently been identified'. He went on to say that there had been about 1,000 deaths from it in Danzig in three or four months.

From 1865 onwards, cases began to be reported in the medical press, and from time to time localized outbreaks occurred in widely scattered places. Some of these early out-breaks were confused with outbreaks of poliomyelitis, which was also on the increase in the early years of the twentieth century. The distinguishing features of the two diseases were, at this time, well known to neurologists, but not so well known to doctors in general. In 1912 cerebrospinal fever and poliomyelitis became notifiable all over the country, and from 1914 to 1918 there was an epidemic of cerebro-spinal fever which was much larger and more widespread than anything which had gone before.

This epidemic of the First World War, which began in the winter of 1914–15, was associated with outbreaks in army camps, particularly those on Salisbury Plain where the first contingent of Canadian troops was quartered. The largest number of cases occurred in the first year (winter 1914–15)

* M. Viesseux, 1805.   † A. Hirsch, 1833–6.

and there was a rapid falling off in subsequent years so that by 1922 annual notifications had reverted to the usual endemic level. In this epidemic the proportion of cases was greater in the services than in the civilian population and the disease was commoner among recruits than among seasoned troops. Glover and others showed that in overcrowded barracks where cases of cerebrospinal fever occurred the appearance of obvious cases of disease was preceded by a rise in the number of healthy carriers of the meningococcus. Sometimes as many as 60 per cent of the troops in a barracks might be harbouring meningococci in the nose and throat whereas the incidence of obvious disease was under 1 per cent.

Between the World Wars the level of incidence remained fairly constant except for a period of activity in the years 1931–3, but in the first winter (1939–40) of the Second World War there was a recrudescence of activity very like that of the first, but on a larger scale. In the year 1940 notifications were 11,185 for civilians and 1,586 for non-civilians.

The chief differences between the epidemics of the two World Wars were that in the first it was the services which were chiefly affected, whereas in the second it was the civilian population, and in the second War the fatality of the disease was much less than it had been because the sulpha drugs, which had come into general use about 1938, were effective in treatment. It is impossible to be quite sure that the epidemic of 1940–3 was much larger than that of 1915–18, because it is likely that ascertainment was more complete in the later period. The difference between the number of cases in the two epidemics is, however, considerable, and is probably too big to be accounted for purely by better diagnosis. In the epidemic of 1914–18 there were about 10,700 cases in England and Wales, whereas in that of 1939–43 there were about 34,700; but in the earlier epidemic 4,136 deaths were among civilians, whereas in the later one the number of deaths was 6,916, representing a much lower case fatality – 20 per cent against 39 per cent. In recent years when meningococcal infections have been endemic rather than epidemic there have been about 1,300 cases a year with about 300 deaths, but these national figures give a rather gloomy picture of the normal fatality of the disease because the deaths usually occur in the atypical cases where the interval between onset and death is only a few hours. Treatment with sulpha drugs and penicillin is effective if started early enough, and in some hospitals the case-mortality is now very low.

The general epidemiological picture of cerebrospinal fever is that of a disease which has been endemic in England for at least a hundred years. There have been two epidemic periods associated with the two World Wars and one lesser epidemic period between them. The last epidemic produced the largest number of cases, but the disease was less fatal than in previous ones because new and successful methods of treatment had been discovered. These have now been improved still more, and if a diagnosis is made quickly and treatment is started at once, patients usually recover. No one knows why epidemics occur, but it looks as though one of the most important factors is the sudden aggregation of young adults in overcrowded barracks which occurs at the beginning of a war. Possibly the importation of unfamiliar strains of meningococcus by troops from abroad may be important, but there is not much evidence of this.

ANTERIOR POLIOMYELITIS
(INFANTILE PARALYSIS)

The popular name infantile paralysis no longer gives a true picture of the usual age incidence of this disease, and so the scientific name anterior poliomyelitis, shortened to poliomyelitis or even 'polio', has come so generally into use that it seems best to call the disease poliomyelitis throughout this section.

Poliomyelitis is an acute infection due to one of the smallest known viruses, or rather to a group of viruses of three main types. The presence of a virus was demonstrated by Landsteiner and Popper* in 1908 by transmission of the

* E. Popper, 1908.

disease to monkeys, and from that time until recently the only method for the detection of most strains of virus was by the inoculation of monkeys. Recently Enders* and his colleagues have succeeded in growing poliomyelitis viruses in cultures of living tissues, a technique which enormously enlarges the scope of the laboratory investigation of the disease.

These viruses have variable effects on different people. They can produce anything from a severe and rapidly fatal illness to a carrier state with no symptoms at all, and it is generally believed that the paralysis which is the distinctive feature of the disease is a comparatively rare result of infection, that the so-called non-paralytic cases far outnumber the paralytic, and that the healthy carriers outnumber the non-paralytic cases. There is, however, some controversy as to the relative proportions of paralytic and non-paralytic cases and of healthy carriers which occur in human populations during epidemics. Some believe that nearly everyone becomes infected at some time in his or her life, whereas others believe that the distribution of the virus is restricted to those in close contact with known cases. Why some develop paralysis when they become infected with the virus whereas others develop a mild febrile illness or no illness at all is unknown, although some people have acquired immunity from single or repeated exposures to infections which have been insufficient to produce disease. In terms of whole populations this factor of silent immunization has been put forward as the explanation for the relative freedom of populations living under primitive conditions from dramatic epidemics of poliomyelitis. The theory is that such populations are, so to speak, 'salted' and so acquire immunity at an early age.

In England, and indeed throughout the world, authentic records of epidemics of poliomyelitis are historically very recent. In England there is a record by Badham† of four cases among children in the small town of Worksop, Nottinghamshire, in the late summer and autumn of 1834, and after that there is a long interval in which no groups of cases were

* J. F. Enders, 1953. † J. Badham, 1834.

reported. Throughout the nineteenth century single cases were often shown at medical meetings and knowledge of the disease gradually became more general, but it was only in the last two decades of the century that groups of cases began to be reported in various parts of the world. In the late summer of 1891 there was a group of cases of paralysis among children in and near the town of Market Rasen in Lincolnshire. This outbreak was described by the medical officer of health in a report which is in the archives of the Local Government Board (now the Ministry of Health). At the time this was thought to be an outbreak of cerebrospinal fever, but there are good reasons for believing that seventeen children who fell ill in the period June to October 1891 really had poliomyelitis. All of them had some degree of paralysis but only two died. This incident is of particular interest because, if it was poliomyelitis and not cerebrospinal fever, this is the first authentic epidemic in England. In the nineties there are several reports from neurologists of small groups of cases, and in the first decade of the twentieth century there are indications that the disease was on the increase in big cities; in 1908 there was an outbreak of eight cases in the village of Upminster, Essex, followed in 1909 by thirty-seven cases in Bristol.

In the years immediately preceding the First World War and particularly in 1911 there was an epidemic wave which affected widely scattered areas in the country. In 1910, for example, the parts chiefly affected were Leicestershire and the north-west coast (Carlisle, etc., and Barrow-in-Furness) whereas in 1911 a widespread prevalence was identified with particularly high incidence in parts of Devon and Cornwall, East Anglia, Westmorland, Birmingham, and in the West Riding of Yorkshire. During the early years of the First World War little was heard of poliomyelitis, but in 1917 the reports of epidemics began again, and thereafter up to 1946 the annual reports of the Chief Medical Officer of the Ministry of Health usually included a record of an epidemic somewhere in the country. Between the World Wars, two years, 1926 and 1938, were outstanding, but even in these the incidence was never on the scale of that experienced in certain other countries, notably in North America and Scandinavia. In the years of high prevalence epidemics were localized in the sense that some counties and cities had dramatic outbreaks, but in addition many other places experienced a slight increase in the number of cases. There were a few exceptions to this general pattern, when only one or two districts had a sharp epidemic in a year while the country as a whole had a year of low incidence. In 1947 the total number of cases notified rose suddenly to 7,776 as compared with the previous highest figure of 1,489 in 1938. But the general pattern of distribution in 1947 was not very different in type from that of previous years. Once again there were centres of epidemic dissemination with an increased prevalence in many other places. The change seems to have been quantitative rather than qualitative. Since 1947 the general level of incidence has been much higher than ever before, and even the years of low prevalence, for example, 1948, have outstripped the years of highest prevalence before the Second World War.

From the historical point of view the most interesting feature about the geographical distribution of poliomyelitis is the tendency for epidemics to recur in certain places sometimes after many years. The reasons why an epidemic in area A in one year should extend into the adjacent area B in the next are not difficult to give, but why area A should have an epidemic in say 1910 and others in 1926 and 1938 is not easy to explain; it is even more difficult to see why, when A has had an epidemic in 1910, B, the area immediately adjacent, should have one perhaps twenty years later. And yet this type of thing seems to have happened oftener than can be explained by pure chance. The problem has been examined in detail for the period between the wars by Professor Bradford Hill,[*] and the author has added a footnote covering the epidemic wave before the First World War. Clearly recurrences in these periods are more impressive as evidence than recent experience, because prevalence has been so widespread since 1947 that it would be possible to find instances of recurrence almost anywhere in the

[*] A. Bradford Hill, 1947.

country. It is, however, interesting that some of the places which were affected early in 1947 had been the scene of considerable epidemics in the past.

Poliomyelitis is no longer a disease of infants in England or indeed in any of the countries of Western civilization. We have somewhat meagre records of the age distribution of cases before 1944, but there can be no doubt that the proportion of older children and adults attacked in recent years has been much higher than it was in the early epidemics. In 1947 about one third of all cases occurred among children under five, about one third in children from five to fourteen, and about one third in persons aged fifteen and over. Children are still more susceptible to the disease, but if adults do contract it they tend to have severe attacks.

In all parts of the world poliomyelitis tends to occur in the warmer months of the year, but of recent years in England cases seem to have occurred more commonly in the colder months than was previously normal, and there have been instances of definite winter epidemics in other countries.

To the student of preventive medicine, poliomyelitis appears, at first sight, to be a thoroughly perverse disease. The greatest epidemics have occurred in countries with relatively high standards of living, and the disease seems to be just as common and as fatal among members of the higher social classes as among those of the lower. It has even been suggested from time to time that members of the higher social classes suffer more, though this view rests on impressions rather than on definite evidence. The usually accepted explanation for this apparent perversity has already been mentioned; it is that the population with relatively low hygienic standards becomes 'salted', whereas that with high standards does not.

From time to time attempts have been made to protect individuals against poliomyelitis by passive or active immunization, but in the 'monkey' era of laboratory work they were completely unsuccessful. Recently the introduction of methods for the culture of virus on living tissues revived interest in the problem of active immunization, and extensive trials of a vaccine prepared from virus killed by formalin have proved the value of the vaccine. The method of control by active immunization is, although not giving complete protection, the only one which seems likely to be effective, because the spread of virus is so often an unseen and therefore uncontrollable affair.

Until 1947 England had been fortunate in its experience of epidemic poliomyelitis in comparison with the Scandinavian countries and with North America, but since then the attack rates have been much higher than ever before, and at present they show no sign of falling to the levels obtaining before 1947.

ENCEPHALITIS LETHARGICA

From the historical point of view epidemic encephalitis lethargica has so far been a nine-days' wonder. Whether it was a disease entirely new to England when it appeared in 1918 is uncertain, but the epidemic which began then and petered out about 1930 was certainly unique in authentic historical records. After the epidemic period a few cases of encephalitis lethargica were still notified every year, but there is considerable doubt whether these were really cases of the same disease or whether they were other forms of encephalitis. It is difficult to distinguish between different kinds of encephalitis from signs and symptoms, and the causal organism of encephalitis lethargica has never been demonstrated, though in other parts of the world several viruses which cause encephalitis have been discovered. Encephalitis lethargica is assumed to be due to a virus because of its analogies with other forms of encephalitis due to viruses and because no larger organism has ever been found.

The chief symptoms and signs noticed in the early cases seen in London and in Sheffield in March and April 1918 were lethargy with paralysis of cranial nerves, particularly of the nerves working the muscles of the eyes, but the symptoms of onset were variable. One of the most distressing features of the disease was that permanent mental changes were apt to occur, and another permanent effect was a condition resembling *paralysis agitans*. In 1918 the disease was reported in fifty-one widely separated districts in England and Wales. The history of notifications is shown in Figure 16. The year 1924 was the year of highest incidence with just over 5,000 notifications and after that there was a gradual decline.

The disease attacked people of all ages and of both sexes, and was commoner in the great centres of population than in rural areas. The first quarter of the year showed the highest number of notifications, with a gradual falling off in the second and third quarters, whereas in the fourth, incidence began to rise again. In most instances there was little evidence of case-to-case infection, but there were striking exceptions to this rule, notably an outbreak in a home for girls at Derby in 1919 in which twelve cases with five deaths occurred among twenty-two residents. There appeared to be no connexion between liability to attack and social conditions.

The epidemiological behaviour of encephalitis lethargica and poliomyelitis exhibits many similarities. The same wide distribution of cases with occasional dramatic localized outbreaks is typical, but the age distribution and the seasonal distribution are quite different. The epidemic form of encephalitis lethargica has now disappeared from the records, but no one can tell whether the story is ended or is to be continued.

11

MALARIA AND YELLOW FEVER

MALARIA and yellow fever are now generally regarded as tropical or at least 'hot country' diseases, but formerly neither disease was confined to the tropics. Malaria had a wide distribution in marshy places throughout the world and was at one time quite important in England. Yellow fever caused some devastating epidemics in the United States in the eighteenth century, of which that in Philadelphia in 1793 is a well-known example. Though it never became very important in England, there was one little outbreak in 1865 which will be described because of its interest as an epidemiological freak.

MALARIA

In the world as a whole malaria is still probably the most important communicable disease, not so much from the aspect of the number of deaths it causes but because of the amount of chronic ill-health which results. In England indigenous malaria is now of no importance at all, but occasionally a single case of the disease, apparently contracted in that country, is reported in the medical press as a curiosity.

The disease is due to a group of protozoa, and the different members of the group produce slightly different symptoms. These protozoa have complicated life histories, and are carried from the infected person to the uninfected by anopheline mosquitoes. Laveran,* a French army surgeon, discovered the protozoa in the blood of infected patients in 1880, and Ross† demonstrated the truth, which had long been suspected, that the protozoa were carried by mosquitoes and that they completed a stage of their complicated

---

* C. A. L. Laveran, 1880. † R. Ross, 1923.

life history within the body of the mosquito. These fundamental discoveries have been enormously important from the point of view of control in tropical countries, and the applied science of malariology has grown up and is concerned with the peculiarities of the different parasites, the ecology of the various anopheline mosquitoes, and the devising of methods for their destruction. From the parochial point of view, it is, however, salutary to remember that these fundamental discoveries had nothing to do with the disappearance of indigenous malaria from England. It had gone before the discoveries were made, as a result of social change which was not directed specifically to the control of malaria.

The early history of malaria in England is lost in a confusion of names. Creighton[*] points out that originally the word 'ague', which later became the popular name for malaria, did not mean a paroxysmal or intermittent fever but merely an acute one. Sydenham[†] frequently uses the term 'ague' to describe various epidemics of febrile diseases, but he makes only one reference to marsh agues. This single reference is in his essay on hysteria, where he interpolates the remark that the blood of a person who has spent two or three days in a locality of marshes and lakes is in the first instance 'impressed with a certain spirituous miasma which produces quartan ague'. It is clear that Sydenham and his contemporaries knew of the endemic 'ague' of marshy districts, but did not regard it as of much importance in comparison with all the other acute fevers which came in epidemics all over England.

We have to wait until Simon's[‡] tenure of office under the Privy Council for any serious attempt to estimate the prevalence of malaria in England. In Simon's sixth report (p. 430) there is a section by Dr G. Whitley on the prevalence of ague and other malarious conditions in the marshy districts of England. He found that the Isle of Sheppey was the chief focus of the disease, but that there was still some in the Fen country and in the marshy districts of the Bristol

* C. Creighton, 1894.   † T. Sydenham, 1676.
‡ John Simon, 1860.

Channel coast near Bridgwater. Except in the Isle of Sheppey it was generally agreed that the amount of disease had declined very much in the twenty years preceding 1860.

By the beginning of the twentieth century indigenous malaria had practically disappeared from England, but the two World Wars aroused fears of a possible recrudescence. In both, large numbers of infected service men arrived back in the country, and mosquitoes which could carry the disease were not uncommon. There was, therefore, a theoretical danger that the disease might become endemic in the marshy districts once again.

YELLOW FEVER

Yellow fever ('Yellow Jack') is caused by a virus carried by certain species of mosquito of which *Aëdes aegypti* is the most important. An attack of the disease confers a long-lasting immunity, and in areas where the disease is endemic the native population has considerable herd immunity. An effective vaccine is now available for protection against the disease. At the present time the disease is confined to the west coast of Africa and to parts of South America, but in the seventeenth, eighteenth, and nineteenth centuries there were many serious epidemics in the ports of the eastern seaboard of North America, extending as far north as Halifax, Nova Scotia (epidemic in 1861). In Europe there were epidemics in Spain and Portugal in the eighteenth and nineteenth centuries, but in England, though ships have often arrived with cases aboard, the disease has spread from a ship to the inhabitants of a port on only one occasion – in Swansea in 1865. This epidemiological curiosity is of sufficient interest to deserve a detailed description: The small barque *Hecla* left Cuba on 26 July 1865. On the voyage several of the crew of ten fell ill, and when she arrived at Swansea on 9 September one seaman was dying and two were convalescent. The *Hecla* was moored next to a small vessel called the *Eleanor* and in the ensuing weeks twenty inhabitants of Swansea and three other members of the crew of the *Eleanor* developed yellow fever. Fifteen of those attacked died. The three members of the crew of the *Eleanor* actually developed the disease at Llanelly. The weather at this time was extremely hot, with temperatures of 80° to 90° F. in the sun and 70° to 80° in the shade.

This unique experience has a little relevance to the present day since the aeroplane has brought the tropics to our doorstep, and it is always a possibility that a person in the incubation stage of yellow fever may arrive and develop the disease in England. We must remember, however, that the Swansea incident is unique and happened long before the part played by mosquitoes in carrying the disease was known. Nowadays strict precautions are taken against the importation of infected mosquitoes and there are also strict rules about the vaccination of travellers. Perhaps the greatest safeguard is the fact that England seems to be a most unfavourable soil for the propagation of epidemics of yellow fever. In the days before much was known about the disease there must have been many undetected importations of 'Yellow Jack', particularly from the West Indies, and yet so far as we know the Swansea outbreak is the only occasion on which the disease spread to the native population and that to a very limited extent.

12

TUBERCULOSIS

TUBERCULOSIS is different from the diseases considered so far in that it has never been 'epidemic' in Britain in the sense of being much more prevalent at one time than at another. It has, however, been an important cause of death throughout the period covered by this book and probably for much longer.

The disease is caused by *Mycobacterium tuberculosis*, discovered by Robert Koch* (1843–1910) in 1882, and two types, the human and the bovine, cause disease in man. Many different organs can be affected, but disease of the lungs is by far the most common form and the easiest to trace in historical records. Laennec (1781–1826), the French physician who invented the stethoscope, recognized the essential unity of tuberculosis of different organs, but the final proof of this unity did not come until Koch's discovery of the tubercle bacillus, and so earlier statistical records of forms of tuberculosis other than respiratory are particularly suspect because of difficulties of classification and confusion with other diseases. In considering the early history of tuberculosis it is better to confine the discussion to disease of the lungs than to attempt a review of all forms of the disease.

PULMONARY TUBERCULOSIS

EARLY HISTORY

The earliest medical books by English physicians about pulmonary tuberculosis (consumption, phthisis) were written in the seventeenth century. In this century Christopher Bennett (1617–55), Thomas Willis (1621–75), Thomas Sydenham (1624–89), and Richard Morton (1639–98) all

* R. Koch, 1882.

either wrote whole books about the disease or devoted chapters to it in general text books. Morton's book, *Phthisiologia*, published in 1688, was the most comprehensive and important of these contributions. Much of the theoretical matter in these books is now out of date, but the descriptions of cases make it clear that the authors were, in the main, writing about tuberculosis of the lungs as we know it today, that the disease was common, and that it was an important cause of death. The Bills of Mortality confirm this, for in most years between fifteen and twenty per cent of all deaths in London were returned under the heading 'consumption'. In plague years, particularly in 1665, the proportion was much lower because the deaths from plague were so many.

Brownlee* reviewed the evidence of the Bills for the whole period 1629–1838 during which causes of death were distinguished. He came to the conclusion that there was an increase in the death rate from pulmonary tuberculosis in London in the eighteenth century which culminated about 1800 and that there was a slow fall in mortality from then on. For the statistical period (1838 onwards) this fall is well authenticated, but the statistics of the earlier period are too doubtful to make it more than a probability. For the country as a whole there are no statistics before 1838, but the growth of towns through immigration from the country districts was going on rapidly, and these new aggregations of susceptible people must have been favourable soil for the spread of the disease. The probability is, therefore, that the rise in mortality, which affected London in the eighteenth century, affected the industrial towns even more, and probably reached its zenith rather later in them than in London.

FROM 1838 TO THE PRESENT DAY

The trend of mortality at all ages

In the first five complete years of registration, the number of deaths assigned to tuberculosis of the lungs was about 60,000 a year out of a total of some 350,000 deaths from all

* J. Brownlee, 1916.

causes. The crude death rate for the quinquennial period 1838–42 was 3,880 per million. There is a gap in the statistical record in the forties because the number of deaths by cause was not abstracted for the years 1843–6. The figures for the years 1851–5 suggest, however, that there was a slow fall in the death rate in the forties. In this quinquennium (1851–5) the total number of deaths averaged about 400,000 a year, and those from tuberculosis of the lungs amounted to about 51,000 a year. The crude death rate for the years

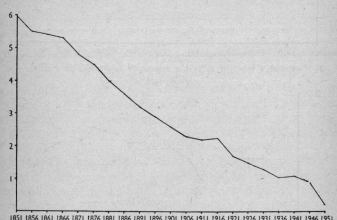

17. *Comparative mortality index, showing trend of respiratory tuberculosis in England and Wales, 1851–1954 (1938 = 1)*

1851–5 was 2,851 per million. The trend of mortality from 1851 to 1954 is shown in Figure 17. This graph is derived from table six of the Registrar-General's *Statistical Review* (Part 1), 1954. In this table he gives comparative mortality indexes for quinquennial periods from 1851–5 to 1931–5, for the four-year period 1936–9, immediately preceding the outbreak of the Second World War, and subsequently for the quinquennial periods 1940–4 to 1950–4. The base year for all comparative mortality indexes is the year 1938 which is taken as unity. Thus mortality in 1851–5 was nearly six times what it was in 1938, whereas in 1950–4 it was 0.25

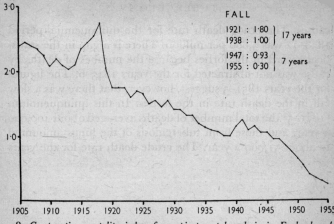

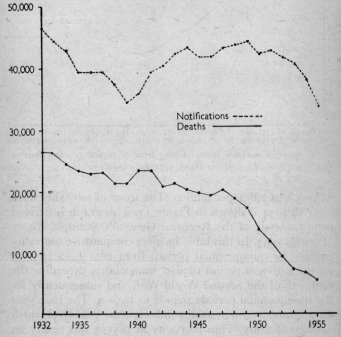

18. *Comparative mortality index for respiratory tuberculosis in England and Wales, 1905–55*

19. *Respiratory tuberculosis. Notifications and deaths in England and Wales, 1932–55*

times that of 1938. The advantage of using the comparative mortality index (C.M.I.) rather than the crude death rate for a long term study is that the C.M.I. makes allowance for the great changes in the age distribution of the population which have taken place in the last hundred years.

The recent trend of annual mortality at all ages is shown in Figure 19 which overlaps the long term graph (Figure 18). The effect of the two World Wars is shown more clearly than in the long term graph, and the prolongation to 1955 brings out the rapidity of the decline of mortality since 1947. The index fell from 1.8 to 1.0 in the seventeen years 1921–38, and from 0.93 to 0.25 in the eight years 1947–55. In this last eight years the new drugs, streptomycin, para-amino-salicylic acid (P.A.S.), and isoniazid (I.N.H.) have come into general use and there have been important advances in surgical treatment.

Incidence

Figure 19 serves as a link between the discussion of mortality and that of incidence. The lower curve is virtually the same as the second half of that shown in Figure 18, but in constructing it the absolute numbers of deaths each year have been plotted instead of the comparative mortality indexes. The total deaths fell from about 27,000 in 1932 to 20,000 in 1947 and 5,837 in 1955. Notifications, on the other hand, have hardly fallen at all. It may be that improved methods of ascertainment, particularly by mass radiography, have had some effect in keeping up the number of notifications, but even allowing for this possibility it seems probable that there has been no decline of incidence comparable to that of mortality.

Changes in the age and sex distribution of mortality

Although mortality at all ages has been falling throughout the statistical period there have been differences in the rate of decline in different age groups. For example the rate of mortality among young women, which has always been higher than that of young men, fell very little between about 1900 and 1932. Recently, however, the death rates of young men and young women have been falling very quickly, much more rapidly than those of middle-aged people, and there has also been a lessening of the difference between young men and young women. Modern methods of treatment are highly successful in young adults but less successful in the middle-aged.

Social Conditions, including occupation

The Registrar-General's studies of occupational mortality have always shown in tuberculosis a rising gradient from social class I (the professional classes) to social class V (unskilled workers). In 1950, according to the analysis of the one per cent sample of the population, the standardized mortality of men in social class V was 2.3 times that of men in social class I.

Within the sub-classes mortality was high among members of the armed forces, dock labourers, and hewers and getters of coal. It was particularly low in agricultural workers. The peculiar dangers of dust containing silicon have long been known, and in the supplement to the thirty-fifth report of the Registrar-General (years 1861–70) Farr drew attention to the fact that steel grinders ran a much greater risk from dust than did those breathing vegetable dusts such as millers. The recognition of this risk has led to a whole series of Acts of Parliament and regulations designed to protect workers in dusty industries and to ensure compensation for those who do contract disease when working in a dusty atmosphere. Though dusts do not themselves cause tuberculosis, they may make the lungs more vulnerable to the effects of infection by tubercle bacillus.

PREVENTION OF TUBERCULOSIS

There are three lines of attack in the prevention of any infectious disease, namely:

1. Stamp out the reservoir of infection.
2. Discourage the vector.
3. Protect the individual.

With tuberculosis, all three methods are of value to us, and, although it is not yet possible to win complete success, the amount of success which can be achieved depends on how well they are applied.

The reservoir of infection in tuberculosis is the so-called 'open case', the patient who has tuberculosis of the lungs and is coughing up live tubercle bacillus. This reservoir may be further considered under two headings:

(a) The known reservoir of infectors, i.e. the known cases of open pulmonary tuberculosis and treatment at clinics and hospitals; in England and Wales the number of these cases in 1955 was estimated to be approximately 20,000.

(b) The unknown reservoir of infectors, i.e. unknown cases of open pulmonary tuberculosis, still at large amongst the general public. It is difficult to give an exact figure for this, but if mass radiography experience is representative of the whole population, there are about 75,000 unsuspected cases of respiratory tuberculosis in the community at any one time or one in every 600 of the population.

Where the patient is known and attending regularly for treatment, much can be done to prevent the spread of the disease. It is not always possible, even with modern drugs, to render him not infectious, but much can be done to minimize the risk by instructing him in methods of personal hygiene and disposal of sputum.

The unknown infector patient is much more dangerous, and the finding of such patients is perhaps the most important task in the preventive service of today. Mass radiography surveys have proved of great value in this respect, but there remains a small group of elderly bronchitics whom it is very difficult to persuade to attend.

Our last line of attack against tuberculosis, protecting the individual, has been much used in this country in recent years. It consists of vaccinating the healthy person with a live but attenuated strain of tubercle bacillus, known as the Bacille Calmette-Guerin (B.C.G.).

This vaccine was brought into experimental use as long ago as 1924, but received a severe setback in 1930 in the Lübeck disaster where, owing to a mistake in culture, children were vaccinated by an active, virulent bacillus and 73 died of tuberculosis.

The vaccine is now manufactured in an isolated laboratory, completely separated from any other building and having its own staff.

The vaccine gives good protection for some five to seven years. In England, it is used to protect all children who have to live in a tuberculous household, all nurses and staff of tuberculosis clinics and hospitals, and, lastly, it is given to school children of fourteen years of age to afford protection in these adolescent years, as it is in the late teens, when these children first go out into the world, that tuberculosis is most likely to develop.

13

THE RELATIVE IMPORTANCE OF THE
DIFFERENT DISEASES AT
DIFFERENT TIMES

THE characters in this book are diseases, and in order that
we may see them in relation to one another at different
periods of history it is interesting to analyse the deaths by
cause in certain years when one or other disease has been
at its zenith. This is a rough and ready method of comparison which introduces a little more precision into the story
than the bare '*magna mortalitas*' of the chroniclers of the
Black Death. As we progress through the centuries the
picture becomes clearer, and the year 1838, when the Bills
of Mortality were replaced by proper registration, is a most
important landmark. From then on the figures are far more
accurate and comprehensive than they had ever been
before.

1665

The year of the Great Plague is the most convenient starting
place, because it marks the end of that period, lasting nearly
300 years, during which plague dominated the scene so
much that other epidemic diseases paled into insignificance
beside it. The complete Bill for 1665 (see Appendix, p. 149)
gives a total of 97,306 burials, 'whereof of the plague'
68,596. The heading which comes next numerically is that
called 'ague and feaver' with 5,257 burials. It seems likely
that some of the deaths really due to plague were returned
under this heading, since the number is considerably swollen
in comparison with the figures of other years. In 1664, for
example, there were 15,453 burials in the Bills and 2,258
of them were ascribed to 'ague and feaver'. In the whole
period of five years 1660–4 there were some 71,000 burials
noted in the Bills – only about 2,000 more than the number

ascribed to plague alone in 1665. Never since then has the mortality from an epidemic disease been so overwhelming. Small wonder that a disease which could cause as many deaths in a year as usually occurred in five years from all causes was an ever-present shadow over the lives of our ancestors, particularly those who lived in London!

1772–1814

The year 1772 is of particular interest because it was the year in which deaths from smallpox in the London Bills reached their zenith of 3,992 (see Figure 7a). The position of smallpox was, however, nothing like that of plague in the seventeenth century because deaths from 'fever', probably chiefly typhus fever, were not far behind, being 3,207 in 1772. The total number of deaths in the year was 26,053, so that smallpox and 'fever' between them accounted for 28 per cent of the total. The nomenclature of diseases in the Bills was in some respects archaic even for the eighteenth century, and this makes it impossible to describe the trend of many diseases. The number of deaths from both smallpox and 'fever' almost certainly declined a little in the last thirty years, and those from smallpox declined rapidly in the early part of the nineteenth century (see Figure 7b). On the other hand, deaths attributed to measles and whooping-cough increased, though it is impossible to be sure whether this was a real increase or due to rather better reporting.

The whole period of the second half of the eighteenth century is of great general interest because it marked the beginning of the rapid growth of population which lasted throughout the nineteenth century and only began to slow down at the end of the first decade of the twentieth. There was no census until 1801, and so earlier statistics of population are to some extent controversial, but between 1750 and 1801 (first census) the population of England and Wales probably increased from about 6½ millions to about 9 millions and that of London from about 675,000 to about a million. It is generally accepted that the increase was due to a decline in the death rate – particularly the death rate in young children – rather than to an increase in the birth rate. Edmonds,* writing in the *Lancet* of 1835–6, made some simple calculations from the Bills of Mortality which show that there was a substantial fall in the mortality of young children in London, and it seems reasonable to suppose that the fall was even greater in the far healthier countryside:

	1730–49	1750–69	1770–89	1790–1809	1810–29
Annual baptisms (average)	15,773	15,370	17,474	19,320	23,896
Annual deaths of children under 5 years old (average)	11,754	9,685	9,003	7,979	7,590
Deaths per cent of baptisms	75	63	52	41	32

The rise in the number of baptisms may seem inconsistent with the statement that there was no great increase in the birth rate in this period, but it must be remembered that London differed from the country as a whole in that it grew not only by natural increase but by immigration from the rest of the country.

From the strictly medical point of view it is not easy to see exactly why the decline of the death rate began when it did. There were no great discoveries in the fields of prevention or of the treatment of diseases. There was, however, a little lightening of the shadows. Throughout the second half of the eighteenth century hospitals and dispensaries for the sick poor were being founded by charitable subscriptions both in London and in the industrial areas which were growing so rapidly. Distinguished physicians like Lettsom, working at the General Dispensary in Aldersgate Street, Clerk of Newcastle, Ferrier of Manchester, and Currie of Liverpool were beginning to penetrate into the slums and to write about the horrors which they found there. In particular they wrote about the prevalence of epidemic typhus which was by this time almost unknown among the more prosperous citizens. Social historians have laid stress on the

* T. R. Edmonds, 1835.

contribution which the doctors made to the reduction of the death rate, but general social causes must have been important too. Throughout the eighteenth century methods of farming were improving rapidly and the reforming land-lords were producing food for the growing populations of the towns on land which had hitherto produced enough for the local inhabitants only. The quality of food was improv-ing because root crops made it possible for farmers to keep their animals throughout the winter instead of killing most of them in the autumn. These fundamental changes must have improved the diet of the poor and any improvement would reduce the general mortality, in particular that of typhus which is pre-eminently a disease of famine. By modern standards the diet of the poor of the cities was still appalling, but we have to compare it with what went before and not with what came after. Although the period of sanitary reform came considerably later, in the second half of the nineteenth century, there were beginnings towards the end of the eighteenth. The sheer discomfort of living in cities with no proper drainage, water supply, or refuse disposal made elementary improvements essential but con-scious efforts to improve the public health by sanitary measures were long delayed. For example, up to 1815 it was illegal to connect the drains from a house to a public sewer and the houses of the rich had cesspools under the basement. Sanitation in the poorer quarters of cities was unspeakably crude. Once again, however, we must make comparisons with what went before and say that there was a little improvement.

1815–48

After 1815, the population continued to grow at a rapid rate, but the rate of growth was already established and there does not appear to have been any outstanding alteration in the birth or death rates. Once the death rate has fallen below the birth rate to any considerable degree a population will continue to grow without any further alteration of rates or even in spite of a degree of adverse change.*

* M. C. Buer, 1926.

In the first half of the nineteenth century there were two main trends influencing social conditions, the one favourable to the public health and the other unfavourable, and the two cancelled one another. The favourable factors were chiefly better feeding and more enlightened medicine; the unfavourable factor, the enormous and uncontrolled growth of the great industrial towns. Social conditions in these new towns tended to be worse than those in London, since many had no form of local government capable of ensuring even the most elementary standards of public hygiene.

So far as individual diseases were concerned the number of smallpox deaths declined considerably in London (see Figure 7b) and probably elsewhere. Deaths from 'fever' declined in London and probably increased in the large ports and industrial towns, particularly in Liverpool which received many Irish immigrants. Typhus was probably the most important fever, but there can be no doubt that there was typhoid too, and in August 1826 Hewett (quoted by Creighton*) of St George's Hospital published an account of ten fatal cases of a fever which was almost certainly typhoid. The common infectious diseases of childhood began to occupy an important place in the London Bills of Mortality and in the writings of medical men in other cities (cf. Watt† in Glasgow).

In 1831 there began the first epidemic of Asiatic cholera, important enough in itself but even more important in its results, because it was the fear of cholera which made people realize how bad sanitary conditions were and so led to the series of Public Health Acts of which that of 1848 was the first.

The events which led up to the Act of 1848 are not strictly relevant to the history of diseases, but mention must be made of the establishment of the General Register Office in 1837 and of Chadwick's‡ *General Report on the Sanitary Condition of the Labouring Population of Great Britain* of 1842. The General Register Office collected the facts about life and death for the whole country and Chadwick's report drove

* C. Creighton, 1894. † R. Watt, 1813.
‡ Sir E. Chadwick, 1837.

them home to many influential people who had little idea of how the other half of the world lived.

1848–75

The year immediately following the first Public Health Act is an interesting one in which to take another look at the prevailing epidemic diseases of London because cholera is shown at its worst. It must be remembered that the Registration Area was much larger than that of the Bills and that the information collected, though still defective, was much more complete. The Registration Area had a population of 2,360,000, and 68,755 deaths were registered in the year. Of these deaths 26,243 were ascribed to the seven principal epidemic diseases:

Cholera	14,125	
Diarrhoea	3,463	(chiefly deaths of infants)
Typhus	2,482	(typhoid included with typhus)
Whooping-cough	2,349	
Scarlatina	2,149	(including diphtheria*)
Measles	1,154	
Smallpox	521	
	26,243	

Some of these figures were understated, as deaths of infants resulting from epidemic diseases were often returned under indefinite causes such as 'convulsions'. The number of births was 72,612 and of deaths among children under five years of age, 24,999, so that if we express the number of deaths under five as a percentage of the births as Edmonds† did for earlier years (see table on p. 133) we arrive at the figure 34 – not very different from the figure for the years 1810–29.

The period between the first Public Health Act of 1848 and the great consolidating Act of 1875 was one of intense activity in the field of preventive medicine. Many men played important parts in the cleansing of the Augean

* It is doubtful whether diphtheria was of any importance at this time.
† T. R. Edmonds, 1835.

stables the growth of cities had created, but three names stand out. Edwin Chadwick (1800–90) was the ruthless administrator, William Farr, the reflective student and research worker, while John Simon (1816–1904) comes somewhere between the two. Chadwick's official life, from his appointment as an Assistant Commissioner of the Poor Law in 1832 to his compulsory retirement from the General Board of Health in 1854, was relatively short, but his achievement was great and his contribution to the future of public health incalculable. Farr was appointed compiler of abstracts to the General Register Office in 1839 and retired in 1879. Thus he was largely responsible for the analysis of the information about life and death in this country for the first forty years of general registration. He supplied the ammunition which Chadwick and Simon used in their war against dirt and disease. Simon was appointed Medical Officer of Health for the City of London in 1847 and from 1855 to 1876 served the various government departments which were successively charged with the care of the public health. Simon's period of office at the Privy Council (1858–72) was his golden age. In spite of the fact that the legal powers of the Privy Council were limited Simon promoted a number of inquiries into the incidence and mortality of diseases in different districts which had an enormous influence in promoting sanitary reform.

In the supplement to the thirty-fifth *Annual Report* of the Registrar-General (1861–70), Farr traced the march of an English generation through life and compared the mortality experience of the 'healthy districts' with that of England as a whole and with that of Liverpool which was then the supreme example of an 'unhealthy district'. His table showing the numbers of children dying under five years of age from various causes is an admirable summary of the relative importance of the principal epidemic diseases in the years 1861–70. The part of Farr's table which relates to epidemic diseases is reproduced on p. 138.

Appalling as the facts revealed in this table were they were not a complete picture. There was another indefinite heading in the table – 'Brain Diseases' – which included a large number of deaths of young children from one of the acute infectious diseases. In the Liverpool district there were 49,840 deaths under this heading. Thus in Liverpool nearly half the children born died before the age of five, and even in the healthy districts just over one-sixth died before that

Table showing the number of deaths of children under five out of 1,000,000 children born alive (1) in the healthy districts, (2) in all England, (3) in the Liverpool district. (Based on the returns for the years 1861–70)

	Healthy Districts	England	Liverpool
Deaths from all causes	175,410	263,182	460,370
Smallpox	602	3,331	5,175
Measles	5,257	11,507	25,514
Scarlatina	11,373	17,959	26,818
Diphtheria	4,184	2,425	3,395
Whooping-cough	9,650	14,424	32,551
Typhus (with enteric and common fever)	2,807	5,401	9,297
Diarrhoea and dysentery	9,354	20,344	51,911
Cholera	399	1,129	4,255
Other zymotic diseases	6,135	10,579	12,092
Total zymotic diseases	49,761	87,099	171,009

(N.B. Zymotic diseases was the term roughly equivalent to the modern term Acute Infectious Diseases.)

age. Farr does not give a detailed table for London, but he gives a summary which shows that the figure for deaths from all causes was 304,518. Thus London came between Liverpool and the whole of England.

Figures for the decennial period provide a good idea of the general level of mortality from epidemic diseases, but they do not show how disastrous were the effects of individual epidemics. In 1863 and 1873, for example, more than 30,000 deaths were ascribed to scarlet fever, and in London alone there were about 6,000 deaths from this disease in 1869 and in 1870. The last epidemic of cholera was in 1865–6. It was smaller than its predecessors and affected chiefly the East

End of London, where the new sewage system was not yet completed. The last great outbreak of classical smallpox occurred in 1871-2, and in the two years there were 42,000 deaths in England and Wales, nearly 10,000 of them in London.

1875-1900

In 1889-92 there was a pandemic of influenza which affected England chiefly in 1891-2. Ever since then influenza has been an important epidemic disease.

After 1872 the death rate of smallpox declined rapidly. Scarlet fever was the most fatal of the common infectious diseases of childhood at the beginning of the period, but at the end of the century measles and whooping-cough came almost equal first, diphtheria second, and scarlet fever last with a death rate less than half that of measles or of whooping-cough.

The death rate, and probably the incidence, of the enteric fevers (typhoid and paratyphoid) declined between 1871 and 1890 and then remained constant until 1900. The decline was probably associated with the improvements which were being made in public water supplies. These improvements in the public health affected the mortality of adults and of older children more than they affected that of babies, and infant mortality in the quinquennium 1895-1900 was even a little higher than in the decennium 1841-50.

In this last quarter of the nineteenth century the new science of bacteriology came into its own and discoveries of micro-organisms which cause disease were announced nearly every year. At first the discovery of the micro-organism which caused a disease seemed likely to lead to the effective control of that disease, but soon it became evident that control was not so easy. The discovery of the existence of healthy carriers or organisms which could produce disease in others made it obvious that, with some diseases, the isolation of those who had obvious symptoms only would never prevent spread.

Studies of immunity which had their origin in Pasteur's work on chicken cholera, anthrax, and rabies were also going on in this period, and in 1890 von Behring* (1854–1917) made an antitoxin which was effective in the treatment of diphtheria.

1900–1914

The decline in the death rate of diphtheria which began in the early part of the twentieth century was probably due largely to the introduction of antitoxin (see Figure 13). The death rate of the enteric fevers which had remained constant from about 1885 to 1900 also began to fall about 1900, and it seems plausible to suppose that this second fall was associated with the greater precision which bacteriology brought to measures of control (see Figure 8).

The greatest change in the trend of mortality in the early twentieth century related, however, to infants. The infant mortality rate had been almost constant at about 150 deaths per thousand live births from the beginning of registration (1838) to 1901, but since then it has declined steadily except for small setbacks in the two World Wars, and in 1954 the rate was 25.4. There are many indefinite causes of death in infancy, and it is, therefore, difficult to make valid generalizations about the causes of this decline, but general improvements in social conditions and better care of infants seem to have been more important than advances in methods of treatment. The reduction in the size of families may have been important, because a school child often brings infectious disease into its home and many infections are more fatal to babies than they are to older children.

In the years immediately preceding the outbreak of the First World War the epidemic diseases which had been important causes of death among older children and adults had become relatively unimportant. Typhus, cholera, and smallpox had virtually disappeared, the enteric fevers were much less common, and scarlet fever, though probably as prevalent as ever, was less fatal. Influenza was, at this time, more a nuisance than a serious cause of death. Although the death rate of diphtheria had declined slowly, it was the

* E. von Behring and Wernicke, 1892.

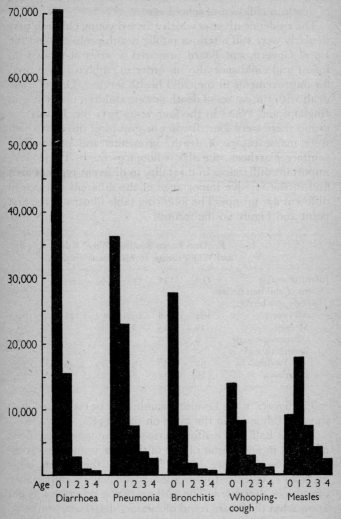

20. *Deaths from diarrhoea, pneumonia, bronchitis, whooping-cough, and measles of children under five in England and Wales, 1911–14 (age 0=infants from birth to first birthday)*

most important of the common infectious diseases as a cause of death in children of school age.

The epidemic diseases which affected young children particularly were still a serious public health problem, and the Local Government Board prepared a series of reports on infant and child mortality in order to emphasize the need for improvements in the child health services. One of these dealt with the causes of death among children under five in England and Wales in the four years 1911–14. In this age group there were four diseases or groups of diseases which were major causes of death: bronchitis and pneumonia, summer diarrhoea, measles, whooping-cough. There were important differences in mortality in different types of area and in the relative importance of the different diseases in different age groups. The following table illustrates the first point and Figure 20 the second:

	England and Wales	Large towns	Smaller towns	Other towns	Rural districts	London
Infant mortality	110	122	113	104	90	108
Deaths of children under 5 per 1,000 births:						
All causes	164	188	167	152	125	164
Measles	12	15	12	10	6	16
Whooping-cough	8	9	8	8	7	8
Bronchitis and pneumonia	32	38	32	29	23	33
Diarrhoea	26	32	28	21	15	30

The figures in the London column may be compared with those of Edmonds in the table on page 133.

Nearly half the deaths ascribed to summer diarrhoea occurred in one season of one of the four years, the exceptionally hot summer of 1911, and so the above table gives an exaggerated impression of the general importance of summer diarrhoea. The authors of the report could not know what the future trend of summer diarrhoea would be, but, in fact, the last great epidemic was that of 1911 (see Figure 10).

The earliest widespread epidemics of poliomyelitis were

reported in the years 1911–13. In this period the disease chiefly attacked children under five, and so its popular name of 'infantile paralysis' was an appropriate one. As a cause of death it was insignificant in comparison with the common infectious diseases, and it was not even mentioned in the report from which the table on p. 142 and Figure 20 were taken. As a cause of crippling, poliomyelitis has been important ever since 1910, and it became relatively more prominent as tuberculosis of bones and joints declined.

1914–18

In the winter of 1914–15 cerebrospinal fever appeared in certain army camps, particularly in those on Salisbury Plain where the first contingent of Canadian troops was quartered. In the First World War the disease affected the services more than civilians, and outbreaks were commoner among recruits than among seasoned troops. The outstanding epidemic of the war years was, however, that of influenza, which began in the early summer of 1918 and reached a climax in the autumn and winter. An exact comparison with the great epidemics of earlier years is impossible, but anyone who lived through it must remember that nearly everyone had the disease. The number of deaths attributed to influenza in the two years 1918–19 was 157,000, but there is no doubt that many deaths really due to influenza were returned under other headings, particularly that of pneumonia. The deaths ascribed to pneumonia were much higher in these two years than in those preceding or following them. Influenza killed at least three times as many people in England and Wales as did the worst epidemic of cholera in 1849, but between 1849 and 1918 the population had increased from about 17 millions to 37 millions. The chief feature of the pandemic of 1918–19 was that all over the world the disease was more fatal to those in the prime of life than it had ever been before or has been since.

In March and April 1918 the first cases of encephalitis lethargica were reported in London and in Sheffield. There had been an epidemic of the disease in Vienna in the war years, but doctors in England only heard about it after the end of the war and were at first puzzled by the bizarre symptoms and signs.

1919–39

The influenza epidemic of 1891–2 was followed by a prolonged rise in the general level of mortality from the disease, and in the years following that of 1918–19 there was a further step-up. The highest rate of the years between the World Wars was recorded in 1929, and after that there was a slow decline of the death rate both in epidemic and in non-epidemic years (see Figure 6).

The death rate from the enteric fevers maintained the steady decline which had begun in 1900. Incidence, however, after a steep fall between 1911 and 1920 showed no consistent trend in the twenties. In the thirties the general level of incidence was lower, but was high in 1936 and 1937 chiefly because of the epidemics of typhoid fever in Bournemouth (1936) and Croydon (1937).

Summer diarrhoea of infants had almost disappeared by 1920, but there was a small rise in the infant mortality from this cause in the hot summer of 1921.

There were interesting differences between the trends of mortality from the common infectious diseases of childhood. At the beginning of the period the death rates of diphtheria, measles, and whooping-cough among children under fifteen were not very different from one another. That of scarlet fever was much lower. By 1939 mortality from measles and whooping-cough had declined so much that diphtheria had become easily the most important of the common infectious diseases, particularly among children of school age. Mortality from scarlet fever had declined still further, and by 1939 the disease was of no importance as a cause of death. From 1911 onwards national statistics of notifications of diphtheria and scarlet fever were collected, and these showed that there was no long term change in the trend of incidence of the two diseases. Measles and whooping-cough were not made notifiable until 1940, and so there are no national statistics of their incidence between the World Wars. It seems probable, however, that the long-term trend of incidence of these two diseases did not change either, and that the decline of their death rates was entirely due to the fact that they became less fatal. Deaths from measles and whooping-cough are usually caused by complications rather than by the

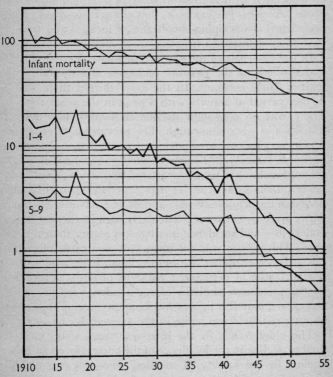

21. *Death rates (all causes) of children in different age groups in England and Wales, 1911–55 (on logarithmic paper to facilitate comparisons between the rates of decline in the different age groups)*

diseases themselves, and the commonest of these fatal complications is broncho-pneumonia. The mortality from broncho-pneumonia also declined greatly between the wars, and the total effect of these favourable trends may be seen in Figure 21 which shows the annual death rates from all causes in different age-groups of childhood from 1911 to 1955. The most prominent peaks on the curves of age-groups 1-4 and 5-9 are in 1918 and were due to influenza. The lesser peaks are most obvious in the curve for age-group 1-4, and were all associated with high prevalence of one or more of the acute infections. For example, that of 1922 was due to high prevalence of whooping-cough and of measles and that of 1929 to epidemics of whooping-cough and influenza.

In the last years of the war cerebrospinal fever declined, and throughout the twenties incidence and mortality remained fairly constant. In the early thirties there was a further period of activity with a peak in the years 1931-2. There was no consistent decline in fatality like that of measles and whooping-cough. The prevalence of encephalitis lethargica rose to a peak in 1924 and then gradually declined. Poliomyelitis occurred throughout the period but the outbreaks were usually scattered and the incidence was never on the same scale as that experienced in the same period in the Scandinavian countries and in North America. There were two years of particularly high incidence – 1926 and 1938 – and incidence in 1938 was higher than that in 1926. This disease was not important as a cause of death, but as other crippling diseases declined, it became an important cause of permanent paralysis of limbs. There are no comprehensive statistics of age-incidence for the inter-war years, but the figures for London suggest that after about 1930 there was a rise in the average age of attack.

The chief trends in the inter-war years were, then, a further decline in the incidence of the enteric fevers; a great decline in the fatality of measles, whooping-cough, and scarlet fever; little change in the incidence or severity of cerebrospinal fever and poliomyelitis.

THE SECOND WORLD WAR AND AFTER

In the years 1940 and 1941 there was a sharp rise in the notifications of paratyphoid fever and a small rise in the death rate from this disease. In the same years cerebrospinal fever had the highest recorded prevalence since that of 1915, and the favourable trend of death rates of infants and children was temporarily reversed. The epidemic of cerebro-spinal fever, unlike that of the First World War, affected the civilian population more than the services. The disease was less fatal than it had been because the sulpha drugs were far more effective than any treatment which had been available before. In 1941 the comprehensive scheme for the immunization of children against diphtheria was inaugurated and in the years since then the disease has almost disappeared.

The later war years were uneventful and the decline of the death rates of infants and children was even more rapid than it had been before the beginning of the war.

In 1946 there were no fewer than fifteen importations of severe smallpox, and in this and the following year there was an increase in the number of cases to 56 in 1946 and 78 in 1947.

The most important event of 1947 was the sudden and unexplained increase in the prevalence of poliomyelitis. At the end of June it became clear that the usual seasonal rise in notifications was much greater than in any previous year and in the week ended 5 July more notifications were received than there had been in the highest week of 1938. The peak of the epidemic came in the week ended 6 September when 708 cases were notified compared with the previous record of 85 cases in a week in October 1938. In the whole year there were about four and a half times as many cases as in 1938. Since the end of June 1947 poliomyelitis had been the most prominent epidemic disease of England. There have been good and bad years but the general level of incidence has been higher than it ever was before and, so far, there is no sign of a consistent downward trend.

Since 1948 the Chief Medical Officer of the Ministry of Health has included in his annual report a short section on the noteworthy outbreaks of epidemic diseases in each year. A rough analysis of these is of interest in that it gives a general picture of the epidemic situation at the present time. In the period there have been two small outbreaks of typhoid fever and three of paratyphoid. Outbreaks of food poisoning caused by one or other of the Salmonellae appear in every report and four were selected for special notice. Severe smallpox occurred three times and mild smallpox once. The other special reports concerned diphtheria and poliomyelitis. It is a sign of the times that individual outbreaks of diphtheria can be singled out for special notice. As recently as 1941 the disease was so common that it would have been impossible for the Chief Medical Officer to select individual outbreaks. The special reports on poliomyelitis relate to districts where prevalence was particularly high in a restricted area in the Isle of Wight in 1950 and at Guildford in 1952.

These then are the diseases which have been of particular concern to the Ministry of Health in recent years. Poliomyelitis is the only one of them which has been epidemic in the country as a whole, though outbreaks of food poisoning have been more common than they should be. The other diseases may be described as rare specimens. Fortunately all of them cause relatively few deaths and all except poliomyelitis can be prevented. The production of a vaccine against poliomyelitis gives promise that in the next few years it may be possible to stop the spread of this disease.

APPENDIX

A general Bill for this present year,

ending the 19 of *December* 1665 according to the Report made to the KINGS most Excellent Majesty.

By the Company of Parish Clerks of *London*, &c.

	Buried	Pla.		Buried	Pla.
St Albans Woodstreet	200	121	St James Dukes place	262	190
St Alhallowes Barking	514	330	St James Garlickhithe	189	118
St Alhallowes Breadst	35	16	St John Baptist	138	83
St Alhallowes Great	455	426	St John Euangelist	9	—
St Alhallowes Honila	10	5	St John Zacharie	85	54
St Alhallowes Lesse	239	175	St Katherine Coleman	299	213
St Alhall. Lumbardstr	90	62	St Katherine Cree-chu.	335	231
St Alhallowes Staining	185	112	St Lawrence Iewrie	94	48
St Alhallowes the Wal	500	356	St Lawrence Pountney	214	140
St Alphage	271	115	St Leonard Eastcheape	42	27
St Andrew Hubbard	71	25	St Leonard Fosterlane	335	255
St Andrew Vndershaft	274	189	St Magnus Parish	103	60
St Andrew Wardrobe	476	308	St Margaret Lothbury	100	66
St Anne Aldersgate	282	197	St Margaret Moses	38	25
St Anne Blacke-Friers	652	467	St Margar. New Fishst	114	66
St Antholins Parish	58	33	St Margaret Pattons	49	24
St Austins Parish	43	20	St Mary Abchurch	99	54
St Barthol. Exchange	73	51	St Mary Aldermanbury	181	109
St Bennet Fynch	47	23	St Mary Aldermary	105	75
St Bennet Grace chur.	57	41	St Mary le Bow	64	36
St Bennet Pauls Wharf	355	172	St Mary Bothaw	55	30
St Bennet Sherehog	11	1	St Mary Colechurch	17	6
St Botolph Billingsgate	83	50	St Mary Hill	94	64
Christs Church	653	467	St Mary Mounthaw	56	37
St Christophers	60	47	St Mary Summerset	342	262
St Clements Eastcheap	38	20	St Mary Stainings	47	27
St Dionis. Back-church	78	27	St Mary Woolchurch	65	33
St Dunstans East	265	150	St Mary Woolnoth	75	38
St Edmunds Lumbard.	70	36	St Martins Iremonger	21	11
St Ethelborough	195	106	St Martins Ludgate	196	128
St Faiths	104	70	St Martins Orgars	110	71
St Fosters	144	105	St Martins Outwitch	60	34
St Gabriel Fen-church	69	39	St Martins Vintrey	417	349
St George Botolphlane	41	27	St Matthew Fridaystr.	24	6
St Gregories by Pauls	376	232	St Maudlins Milkstreet	44	22
St Hellens	108	75	St Maudlins Oldfishstr.	176	121

	Buried	Pla.		Buried	Pla.
St Michael Bassishaw	253	164	St Olaves Iewry	54	32
St Michael Cornehill	104	52	St Olaues Siluerstreet	250	132
St Michael Crookedla.	179	133	St Pancras Soperlane	30	15
St Michael Queenehi.	203	122	St Peters Cheape	61	35
St Michael Querne	44	18	St Peters Corne-hill	136	76
St Michael Royall	152	116	St Peters Pauls Wharfe	114	86
St Michael Woodstreet	122	62	St Peters Poore	79	47
St Mildred Breadstreet	59	26	St Stevens Colemanst	560	391
St Mildred Poultrey	68	46	St Stevens Walbrooke	34	17
St Nicholas Acons	46	28	St Swithins	93	56
St Nicholas Coleabby	125	91	St Thomas Apostle	163	110
St Nicholas Olaues	90	62	Trinitie Parish	115	79
St Olaves Hart-streete	237	160			

Buried in the 97 Parishes within the walls, 15207
Whereof, of the Plague, 9887

	Buried	Pla.		Buried	Pla.
St Andrew Holborne	3958	3103	St George Southwark	1613	1260
St Bartholmew Great	493	344	St Giles Cripplegate	8069	4838
St Bartholmew Lesse	193	139	St Olaves Southwark	4793	2785
St Bridget	2111	1427	St Saviours Southwark	4235	3446
Bridewell Precinct	230	179	St Sepulchres Parish	4509	2746
St Botolph Aldersgate	997	755	St Thomas Southwark	475	371
St Botolph Algate	4926	4051	Trinity Minories	168	123
St Botolph Bishopsgate	3464	2500	At the Pesthouse	159	156
St Dunstans West	958	665			

Buried in the 16 Parishes without the Walls   41351

Whereof, of the Plague   28888

	Buried	Pla.		Buried	Pla.
St Giles in the Fields	4457	3216	St Magdalens Bermon.	1943	1363
Hackney Parish	232	132	St Mary Newington	1272	1004
St James Clarkenwel	1863	1377	St Mary Islington	696	592
St Katherines Tower	956	601	St Mary Whitechap.	4766	3855
Lambeth Parish	798	537	Redriffe Parish	304	210
St Leonards Shorditch	2669	1949	Stepney Parish	8598	6583

Buried in the 11 out-Parishes, in Middlesex and Surrey   28554

Whereof, of the Plague   21420

	Buried	Pla.		Buried	Pla.
St Clement Danes	1969	1319	St Mary Sauoy	303	198
St Paul Covent Garden	408	261	St Margaret Westmin.	4710	3742
St Martin in the Field	4804	2883	*Thereof at the Pesthouse*	—	156

APPENDIX

Buried in the 9 Parishes in the City and Liberties of Westminster	12194
Whereof, of the Plague	8403

The Total of all the Christnings	9967
The Total of all the Burials this year	97306
Whereof, of the Plague	68596

Diseases and Casualties this year.

Abortive and Stilborne	617	Headmouldshot & Mouldfallen	14
Aged	1545	Jaundies	110
Ague and Feaver	5257	Impostume	227
Appoplex and Suddenly	116	Kild by several accidents	46
Bedrid	10	Kings Evill	86
Blasted	5	Leprosie	2
Bleeding	16	Lethargy	14
Bloudy Flux, Scowring & Flux	185	Livergrowne	20
Burnt and Scalded	8	Meagrom and Headach	12
Calenture	3	Measles	7
Cancer, Gangrene and Fistula	56	Murthered, and Shot	9
		Overlaid and Starved	45
Canker, and Thrush	111	Palsie	30
Childbed	625	Plague	68596
Chrisomes and Infants	1258	Plannet	6
Cold and Cough	68	Plurisie	15
Collick and Winde	134	Poysoned	1
Consumption and Tissick	4808	Quinsie	35
Convulsion and Mother	2036	Rickets	557
Distracted	5	Rising of the Lights	397
Dropsie and Timpany	1478	Rupture	34
Drowned	50	Scurvy	105
Executed	21	Shingles and Swine pox	2
Flox and Smal Pox	655	Sores, Ulcers, broken and bruised Limbes	82
Found dead in streets, fields, &c.	20	Spleen	14
French Pox	86	Spotted Feaver and Purples	1929
Frighted	23	Stopping of the Stomack	332
Gout and Sciatica	27	Stone and Strangury	98
Grief	46	Surfet	1251
Griping in the Guts	1288	Teeth and Worms	2614
Hangd & made away themselves	7	Vomiting	51
		Wenn	1

$$
\text{Christned}
\left\{
\begin{array}{ll}
\text{Males} & 5114 \\
\text{Females} & 4853 \\
\text{In all} & 9967
\end{array}
\right\}
$$

$$
\text{Buried}
\left\{
\begin{array}{ll}
\text{Males} & 48569 \\
\text{Females} & 48737 \\
\text{In all} & 97306
\end{array}
\right\}
$$

Of the Plague   68595

Increased in the Burials in the 130 Parishes and at the Pest-house this year   79009

Increased of the Plague in the 130 Parishes and at the Pest-house this year   68590

BIBLIOGRAPHY

1. BADHAM, J. *London Medical Gazette*, 15 (1834), 215.
2. BAILLOU, of Paris. 1578. Cited by Creighton, *see* 17.
3. BARRET-HAMILTON, G. E. H., and HINTON, M. H. C. *History of British Mammals*. London (Gurney & Jackson), 1910–21.
4. BATEMAN, Thomas. *Reports on the Diseases of London*. 1819.
5. BEHRING, E. von, and WERNICKE. *Dtsch. Med. Wschr.*, 39 (1892), 873.
6. BORDET, J., and GENGOU, O. *Ann. Inst. Pasteur*, 20 (1906), 731.
7. BRADLEY, W. H., MASSEY, A., LOGAN, W. P. D., SEMPLE, A. B., BENJAMIN, B., GRIST, N. R., and HOPE SIMPSON, R. E. Discussion – 'Influenza, 1951'. *Proc. Royal Society of Medicine*, xliv (1951), 789–801.
8. BROWNLEE, J. 'The History of the Birth and Death Rates in England and Wales, taken as a whole from 1570 to the present time.' *Public Health* (1916), 211–22, 228–38.
9. BUDD, W. *Typhoid Fever*. London, 1873.
10. BUER, M. C. *Health, Wealth, and Population in the Early Days of the Industrial Revolution*. London (Routledge), 1926.
11. BULSTRODE, H. T. 'Report on Suspected Pneumonic and Bubonic Plague in East Suffolk and on the Prevalence of Plague in Rodents in Suffolk and Essex.' *Reports and Papers on Suspected Cases of Human Plague in East Suffolk and on an Epizootic of Plague in Rodents* (Great Britain, Local Government Board), Vol. I (1911).
12. BURNET, F. M. *Principles of Animal Virology*. New York (Academic Press), 1944.
13. CAIUS, John. *A Boke, or Counseill against the Disease called the Sweate, or Sweatyng Sicknesse*. London, 1552.
14. CHADWICK, Sir Edwin. *General Report on the Sanitary Conditions of the Labouring Population of Great Britain*. London (H.M. S.O.), 1837.
15. CLEMOW, F. *Lancet*, (20 January 1894).
16. CLOWES, William. *A Short and Profitable Treatise on the case of the Disease Called* Morbus Gallicus *by Unctions*. London, 1579.
17. CREIGHTON, C. *A History of Epidemics in Britain*. Cambridge University Press, 1894.

18. DEFOE, D. *Journal of the Plague Year.* 1722.

19. DICK, G. F., and DICK, G. H. *Journal of American Medical Assoc.*, 82 (1934), 265.

20. EDMONDS, T. R. 'The Diminution of the Mortality of Infants in England.' *Lancet*, Vol. I, 1835.

21. ENDERS, J. F. *Proc. Soc. Exp. Biol., New York*, 82 (1953), 100.

22. FARR, W. *Annual Reports of the Registrar-General.* 1861–70.

23. FOSTER, M. G. 'Sweating Sickness in Modern Times.' From *Contributions to Medical and Biological Research Dedicated to Sir William Osler in honour of his seventieth birthday.* New York (Paul B. Hoeber), 1919.

24. FOTHERGILL, J. *An account of the Sore Throat Attended with Ulcers.* London, 1748.

25. GOODALL, Charles. *Book on History of Infectious Diseases.* 1661.

26. GRAUNT, John. *Observations on Bills of Mortality.* 1662. Quoted by Creighton (*see* 17).

27. GREENHOW, E. H. *Deaths by Causes in Different Areas worked under Simon.*

28. GREENWOOD, L. H. *Epidemics and Crowd Diseases.* Williams and Norgate, 1935.

29. HANSEN, G. H. A. *Norsk Mag. Lacquidinsk.* 1874.

30. HARRIS, Walter. *Acute Diseases of Infants.* London, 1689.

31. HEBERDEN, W. 'The Mortality of London.' *Med. Trans. Coll. Physicians of London.* Vol. 4 (1813), 103.

32. HILL, A. Bradford. 'Statistics in the Medical Curriculum.' *B.M.J.*, Vol. II (1947), 366.

33. HIRSCH, August. *Handbuch der historisch-geographisch Pathologie*, 1881. English Translation by C. Creighton, 1833–6.

34. HOME, F. *An Enquiry into the Nature, Cause, and Cure of the Croup.* Edinburgh, 1765.

35. HUXHAM, John. *An Essay on Fevers.* 1755.

36. JENNER, Edward. *An Inquiry into the Causes and Effects of Variolae Vaccinae.* 1798.

37. JENNER, Sir William. *Lectures and Essays on Fevers and Diphtheria, 1847–79.* London, 1893.

38. KOCH, R. *Berl. Klin. Wschr.* 19 (1882), 221.

39. LAVERAN, C. A. L. 'Un nouveau parasite trouvé dans le sang de plusieurs malades atteints de fièvre palustre.' *Bull. Soc. Med. Hop.* (Paris), xvii (1880), 158–64.

40. LETTSON, John C. *Medical Memoirs of the General Dispensary in London.* April 1773 to March 1774.

41. LISTON, W. Glen. 'Milroy Lectures on the Plague.' *B.M.J.*, I (1924), 900, 950, 997.

42. LÖFFLER, F. *Mitt. Reichsgesundheilsamt* 2 (1884), 421.

43. MINISTRY OF HEALTH. (a) *Reports on Public Health and Medical Subjects* (H.M.S.O.), No. 81, 1937. (b) *Annual Report*, 1952.

44. NICOLLE, C., CONOR, A., and CONSEIL, E. *Annals of the Institut Pasteur*, 25 (1911), 97.

45. OSLER, W. *Principles and Practice of Medicine*. 1920.

46. PENNANT, T. *British Zoology* (4 vols.). London (White), 1776-7.

47. PEPYS, S. *Pepys's Diary*, 1825. Deciphered by the Rev. John Smith, 1659-1699.

48. POPPER, E. *Expir. therap.* 2 (1908), 377.

49. ROCHE-LIMA, H. da. *Berl. Klin. Wschr.* 53 (1916), 567.

50. ROLLESTON, J. D. *History of Acute Exanthematous*. London (Heinemann), 1937.

51. ROSS, R. *Memoirs with a full account of the Great Malaria Problem and its Solution*. London (J. Murray), 1923.

52. SIMON, Sir John. *Report on the Last Two Cholera Epidemics of London as affected by the Consumption of Impure Water*. 1856. *Second Report* (for 1859) *by the Medical Officer of the Privy Council*. London, 1860.

53. SMITH, W., ANDREWES, C. H., and LAIDLOW, P. P. *Lancet*, II (1933), 66.

54. SNOW, John. *On the Mode of Communication of Cholera*. 1849.

55. SYDENHAM, T. *Observations Medicae* – 3rd ed. 1676. English translation by R. G. Latham.

56. THOMPSON, T. *Account of Varioloid Epidemic in Scotland*. 1820. *Annals of Influenza*. London (Sydenham Society), 1852.

57. TREVELYAN, G. M. *English Social History*. 1942.

58. VIESSEUX, M. 'Sur la maladie qui a régné à Genève au printemps de 1805.' *J. Med. Chir. Pharm.* (Paris), 1805.

59. WATT, Robert. *A Treatise on the Nature, History, and Treatment of Chincough, to which is subjoined an Inquiry into the Relative Mortality of the Principle Diseases of Children*. Glasgow, 1813.

60. WEICHSELBAUM, A. *Fortschr. Med.* 5 (1887), 573.

61. WILLAN, R. *Description and Treatment of Cutaneous Diseases*. 1798-1808.

62. WILLIS, Thomas. *Diatribe Duae Hogae*. 1659.

63. WOODVILLE, M. *Reports of a Series of Inoculations for the Variolae Vaccinae or Cowpox*. London (J. Phillips), 1799.

INDEX